Spurgeon's Color Atlas of
Large Animal Anatomy:
The Essentials

T0097513

Spurgeon's Color Atlas of
Large Animal Anatomy:
The Essentials

Thomas O. McCracken, MS
Former Associate Professor of Anatomy
College of Veterinary Medicine and Biomedical Sciences
Colorado State University
Vice President for Product and Development
Visible Productions LLC
Fort Collins, Colorado

Robert A. Kainer, DVM, MS
Professor Emeritus of Anatomy
College of Veterinary Medicine and Biomedical Sciences
Colorado State University
Fort Collins, Colorado

Thomas L. Spurgeon, PhD
Late Associate Professor of Anatomy
College of Veterinary Medicine and Biomedical Sciences
Colorado State University
Fort Collins, Colorado

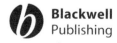 **Blackwell**
Publishing

Blackwell Publishing Professional
2121 State Avenue, Ames, Iowa 50014, USA

Orders:	1-800-862-6657
Office:	1-515-292-0140
Fax:	1-515-292-3348
Web site:	www.blackwellprofessional.com

Blackwell Publishing Ltd
9600 Garsington Road, Oxford OX4 2DQ, UK
Tel.: +44 (0)1865 776868

Blackwell Publishing Asia
550 Swanston Street, Carlton, Victoria 3053, Australia
Tel.: +61 (0)3 8359 1011

Authorization to photocopy items for internal or personal use, or the internal or personal use of specific clients, is granted by Blackwell Publishing, provided that the base fee is paid directly to the Copyright Clearance Center, 222 Rosewood Drive, Danvers, MA 01923. For those organizations that have been granted a photocopy license by CCC, a separate system of payments has been arranged. The fee codes for users of the Transactional Reporting Service are ISBN-13: 978-0-6833-0673-6/2006.

First edition

Library of Congress Cataloging-in-Publication Data
McCracken, Thomas O.
        Spurgeon's color atlas of large animal anatomy : the essentials /
    Thomas O. McCracken, Robert A. Kainer, Thomas L. Spurgeon
        p. cm.
    ISBN 978-0-6833-0673-6
    1. Veterinary anatomy Atlases.   I. Kainer, Robert A.   II. Title.
SF7613M35 1999
636.089'1—dc21   99-20525
                                                                         CIP
Printed and bound in USA by Quad/Graphics
SKY10063009_122023

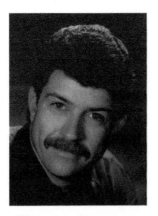

Thomas Spurgeon

TO OUR COLLEAGUE AND FRIEND

Dr. Thomas L. Spurgeon, exceptionally well-trained anatomist, superb teacher, and educational innovator, devoted his professional life to the advancement of anatomic education through scientific investigation and the dissemination of anatomic knowledge.

Following service to his country in the United States Air Force, Thomas L. Spurgeon entered college. Upon completion of his doctorate in anatomy in the School of Veterinary Medicine at the University of California-Davis, Dr. Spurgeon accepted a faculty position in the College of Veterinary Medicine at Washington State University. His record as an excellent anatomist at that institution led to a position in the College of Veterinary Medicine and Biomedical Sciences at Colorado State University.

His broad knowledge of both human and veterinary anatomy was utilized fully at Colorado State. Students requiring courses in basic human anatomy as well as those majoring in veterinary medicine and various animal sciences profited from the instruction provided by this well-rounded anatomist who possessed outstanding pedagogic skill. His expertise was equally appreciated by the graduate students he mentored, particularly those in the biomedical illustration program.

Dr. Spurgeon, a pioneer in the computer-assisted instruction of anatomy, was continually seeking new methods of presentation. He and his colleague and close friend, Thomas O. McCracken, conceived the unique anatomic presentation used in this atlas.

Tragically, Dr. Spurgeon's untimely death in an automobile accident in 1997 brought a halt to his brilliant career. Dr. Spurgeon's devoted sons, Aaron and Kyle, are indeed proud of their father's accomplishments. Countless students mourn the passing of a man who, as teacher and friend, contributed so much to their lives.

ACKNOWLEDGMENTS

Many talented individuals contributed to the production of *Spurgeon's Color Atlas of Large Animal Anatomy: The Essentials.* Foremost among them were the artists, Conery Calhoon, Molly Babich, Gale Mueller, and Sandra Mullins, who colored Thomas McCracken's original drawings of anatomic specimens. They employed manual and digital techniques to reproduce the subtle colors of tissues and organs.

Consultants, who authored plates drawn by Thomas McCracken, selected clinical conditions and husbandry applications based on their anatomic significance. The consultants were Dr. Gayle Trotter for the horse; Dr. Frank Garry for the ox; Dr. Joan Bowen for the sheep and goat; Dr. LaRue Johnson for the llama and alpaca and the swine; and Dr. John Avens for the chicken. These specialists reviewed the plates on the various species, enhancing the accuracy of the presentations. Their contributions are gratefully acknowledged.

Carroll Cann, Executive Editor of Teton-New Media, was an enthusiastic supporter of the concept of the atlas. We thank him for his suggestions and encouragement.

Special thanks are due the late Dr. Patricia Brooks who supported her husband, Dr. Spurgeon, and frequently assisted him in his work. She, too, was a contributor to this atlas.

We greatly appreciated the reliable assistance of Dennis Madden, pathology technician in the College of Veterinary Medicine and Biomedical Sciences at Colorado State University. His procurement of specimens and his dissection skills were essential to the production of this atlas.

We thank Mark Goldstein for a student's viewpoint. His assistance with compilation of the index and his review and comments on the plates were most helpful.

We are grateful to Dr. Michael Smith from the School of Veterinary Medicine at Ross University for his careful review of the final proofs. His knowledge of anatomy, his fine teaching skills, and his critical eye well qualified him for this arduous task.

Acknowledgment is due the Department of Anatomy and Neurobiology and the Department of Clinical Sciences at Colorado State University for the use of their facilities and for providing living animals, skeletons, embalmed specimens, and necropsy specimens. Dr. Robert Lee prepared and was most helpful in providing anatomic specimens. We acknowledge the kindness of exhibitors at the National Western Stock Show and Midnight Valley Friesens for permission to photograph their animals.

We thank Alpine Publications, Inc. of Loveland, Colorado, for permission to use drawings from our book, *Horse Anatomy, A Coloring Atlas.* Permission from Pfizer Animal Health Group to use drawings of the chicken's anatomy from *Anatomical Atlas* is also appreciated.

CONTENTS

SECTION 1   THE HORSE *(Equus caballus)*

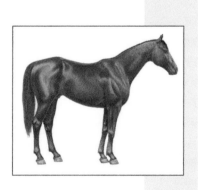

SECTION 2   THE OX *(Bos taurus,* also *Bos indicus)*

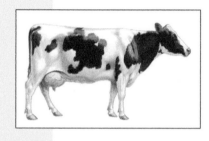

SECTION 3   THE SHEEP *(Ovis aries)*

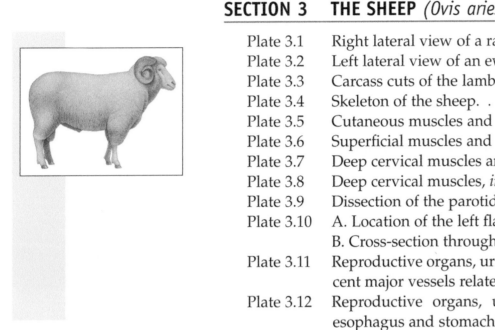

SECTION 4   THE GOAT *(Capra hircus)*

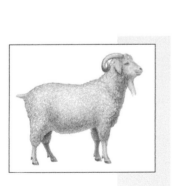

SECTION 5   THE LLAMA AND ALPACA *(Lama glama and Lama pacos)*

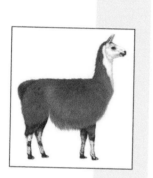

SECTION 6   THE SWINE *(Sus scrofa domesticus)*

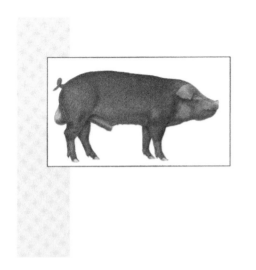

SECTION 7   THE CHICKEN *(Gallus gallus domesticus)*

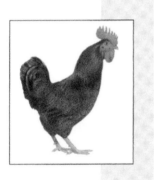

INTRODUCTION

S*purgeon's Color Atlas of Large Animal Anatomy: The Essentials* is not a complete, detailed anatomic atlas. Instead, it presents topographic relationships of the major organs of the horse, ox, sheep, goat, llama, alpaca (a smaller species with long, lustrous hair), swine, and chicken in a simple yet technically accurate format. As an important food animal, the chicken is included with the large domestic animals in this atlas. Throughout the *Atlas*, most male and female of a given species are on facing pages. The majority of the plates contain information on the entire body. Some plates are confined to a region; a few contain organs isolated from the rest of the body. Whereas most systems (e.g., digestive and reproductive) are presented for each animal, other systems are included only for some species to illustrate general anatomic patterns. Structures common to the various animals are labeled several times; other structures are labeled on only one or two species, usually emphasizing specific anatomy (the anatomy peculiar to a certain species). Animal specialists authored plates illustrating selected clinical or husbandry applications that reflect the anatomy of the organs involved.

The *Atlas* is intended for use by individuals at different stages of their education, serving as a survey of the specific anatomy of the different animals. Advanced 4-H club members, high school vocational agriculture students, and college students studying veterinary medical technology, veterinary medicine, animal science, and wildlife biology can use this *Atlas* as an introduction to the anatomy of common farm animals. The *Atlas* can also serve as a reference for horse breeders and trainers, as well as livestock and poultry producers. It will provide a quick review for persons with previous training in anatomy and will be an invaluable aid for the professional—e.g., a veterinarian or animal scientist—in explaining to a client some aspect of anatomy that pertains to an animal's condition and needs.

The following introductory pages provide the reader with a background in nomenclature and anatomic orientation.

ANIMAL CLASSIFICATION

The horse (*Equus caballus*) is classified as an odd-toed ungulate (hoofed mammal) in the order Perissodactyla, suborder Hippomorpha, and family Equidae. Members of this family are termed equids. "Equine" is an adjective. Equine characteristics include the grouping of limb muscles close to the trunk with tendons extending over long third metacarpal and metatarsal bones to the digits, providing leverage for sustained, rapid locomotion. Because this leverage arrangement does not develop great force, the heavy draft horse must rely on body weight to perform pulling tasks. Another equine characteristic is the horse's extensive large intestine, the site of final microbial digestion and absorption of nutrients.

Cloven-hoofed ungulates that walk on their third and fourth digits are in the order Artiodactyla. Domestic ungulates in the suborder Ruminantia include those in the family Bovidae, subfamily Bovinae—the ox (*Bos taurus*) and zebu (*Bos indicus*)—and subfamily caprinae, the sheep (*Ovis aries*) and goat (*Capra hircus*). The noun "bovids" (after Bovidae) is usually reserved for cattle, bison, yak, and water buffalo; sheep are ovids and goats are caprids, named according to each genus. Adjectives end in -ine: bovine, ovine, and caprine, respectively.

The llama (*Lama glama*) and alpaca (*Lama pacos*) are cud-chewing artiodactyls from South America called camelids, named after the family Camelidae in the suborder Tylopoda. South American camelids are also called lamoids. Both ruminants and camelids have large, compartmented stomachs essential for the microbial digestion of cellulose. Feed is more finely divided by rumination, a physiologic sequence of regurgitation of stomach contents, remastication (chewing), and redeglutition (swallowing).

Swine (pigs are young; hogs are mature) are artiodactyls in the suborder Suiformes, family Suidae. Domestic swine (*Sus scrofa domesticus*) are descended from the European wild boar with some input from the smaller *Sus indica* from China. The adjective "porcine" is derived from the Latin *porcinus*, from porcus, a hog. Reflecting its omnivorous diet, the swine's digestive tract is somewhat simpler than those of ruminating animals.

The chicken or domestic fowl (*Gallus gallus domesticus*) is classified with other comb-bearing gallinaceous birds in the order Galliformes. Descended from the Red Junglefowl of southeast Asia, the chicken is in the family Phasianidae.

GENERAL TERMINOLOGY

With some exceptions, particularly for most muscles wherein traditional Latin names are used, the terminology in this *Atlas* conforms to English translations of Latin terms in the *Nomina Anatomica Veterinaria (N.A.V.)*, 3rd ed., 1983. There are some departures from N.A.V., however. For example, according to N.A.V., the hoof includes the underlying corium (dermis) with the horny epidermis, whereas in common usage hoof refers only to the horny epidermal structure. In compliance with the intent of N.A.V., nomenclature will be consistent for all species. Common terms and meat-packing terms are used on some plates. Abbreviations for organs in this *Atlas* include: a, artery; b, bone; j, joint; lig., ligament; ln, lymph node; m, muscle; n, nerve; v, vein. Double letters indicate the plural form of these words (e.g., aa, arteries). Positional and directional terms, body planes, and the extent of body cavities are used to indicate the location of parts of the body and functional changes in position. The extent of diseased regions is defined using this anatomic terminology.

POSITIONAL AND DIRECTIONAL TERMS

The following terms are illustrated on the accompanying drawing of a horse. **Dorsal** and **ventral** are opposite terms indicating relative locations toward the back (L., dorsum) or belly (L., venter). Above the knee (carpus) and hock (tarsus) and from the belly to the back, a structure located closer to the cranium (skull case) is **cranial** to another structure, and a structure located toward the tail (L., cauda) is **caudal** to another. On the head, the term **rostral** indicates a structure closer to the nose (L., rostrum).

Proximal indicates a location toward the attached end of a limb; **distal** indicates a location toward the free end of a limb, that is, further from the trunk. Distal to and including the carpus, **dorsal** replaces cranial; **palmar** replaces caudal. Distal to and including the hock, dorsal replaces cranial, but **plantar** replaces caudal.

On a frontal view of the distal end of a limb, notice that an **axial** structure is located toward the **axis.** An **abaxial** structure is located away from it.

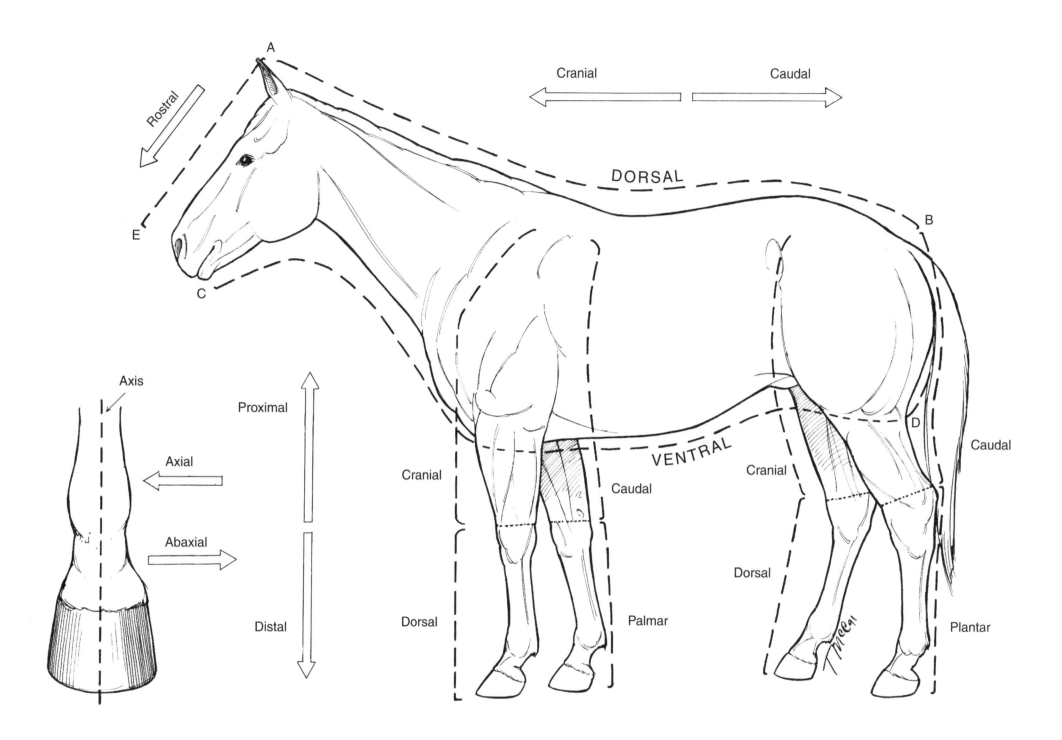

Cranial

Caudal

DORSAL

Rostral

A

B

E

C

VENTRAL

D

Caudal

Axis

Proximal

Cranial

Caudal

Cranial

Axial

Abaxial

Distal

Dorsal

Palmar

Dorsal

Plantar

BODY PLANES

Drawings of a horse are used to illustrate body planes. The **median plane** (L., medius, middle) divides the animal body into right and left halves. A **sagittal plane** (L., sagitta, arrow) is any plane parallel to the median plane. **Medial** and **lateral** (L., latus, side) are directional terms relative to the median plane. Medial structures are located closer to the median plane. Lateral structures lie away from the median plane, that is, toward the side. A **transverse plane** passes through the head, trunk, or limb perpendicular to the part's long axis. A **dorsal plane** (also called a **frontal plane**) is a longitudinal plane that passes through the body parallel to its dorsal surface at right angles to the median plane.

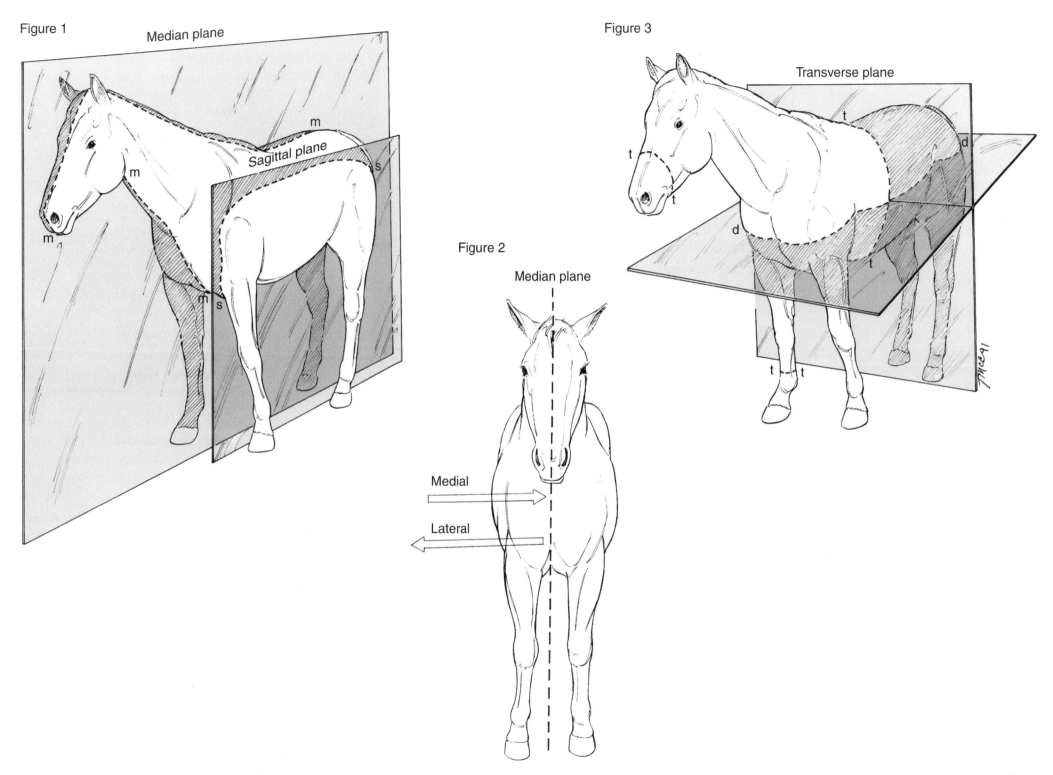

Figure 1

Median plane

m

m

m

m s

Sagittal plane

s

Figure 2

Median plane

Medial

Lateral

Figure 3

Transverse plane

t

t

t

d

d

t

t

t

BODY CAVITIES AND MEMBRANES

A diagrammatic drawing of a mare's trunk illustrates the **thoracic, abdominal,** and **pelvic cavities** and the serous membranes—**peritoneum, pleura,** and **pericardium**—that line the cavities and suspend organs.

The peritoneum consists of three continuous parts. The **parietal peritoneum** (L., paries, wall) lines the abdominal cavity and the cranial part of the pelvic cavity. **Connecting peritoneum** reflects from the parietal peritoneum and suspends organs in a double fold containing vessels and nerves as it extends to an organ. The connecting peritoneum is indicated by mes- (G., mesos, middle) plus the Latin or Greek name of the organ. An example is mesentery: mes- plus G., enteron, small intestine. Peritoneal ligaments suspend and support—e.g., the falciform ligament of the liver. **Visceral peritoneum** is continuous with connecting peritoneum, encircling a viscus (Latin for a large, internal organ; plural, **viscera**).

The musculomembranous **diaphragm** is covered with peritoneum on its abdominal surface and pleura on its thoracic surface.

The **pleurae** are two continuous serous membranes, each forming a pleural sac. The **parietal pleura** lines each half of the thoracic cavity. **Mediastinal pleura** is connecting pleura on each side enclosing the **mediastinum**, a space containing the heart, esophagus, trachea, blood vessels, lymph nodes and ducts, thymus, nerves, and adipose tissue. **Visceral pleura** covers each lung.

The **pericardium** is the heart sac. **Visceral pericardium** (also called epicardium) covers the heart and reflects around the base of the heart and great vessels to become continuous with the **parietal pericardium**.

The serous cavities—**peritoneal cavity, pleural cavity,** and **pericardial cavity**—are potential spaces between parietal and visceral membranes containing lubricating serous fluids named for each cavity.

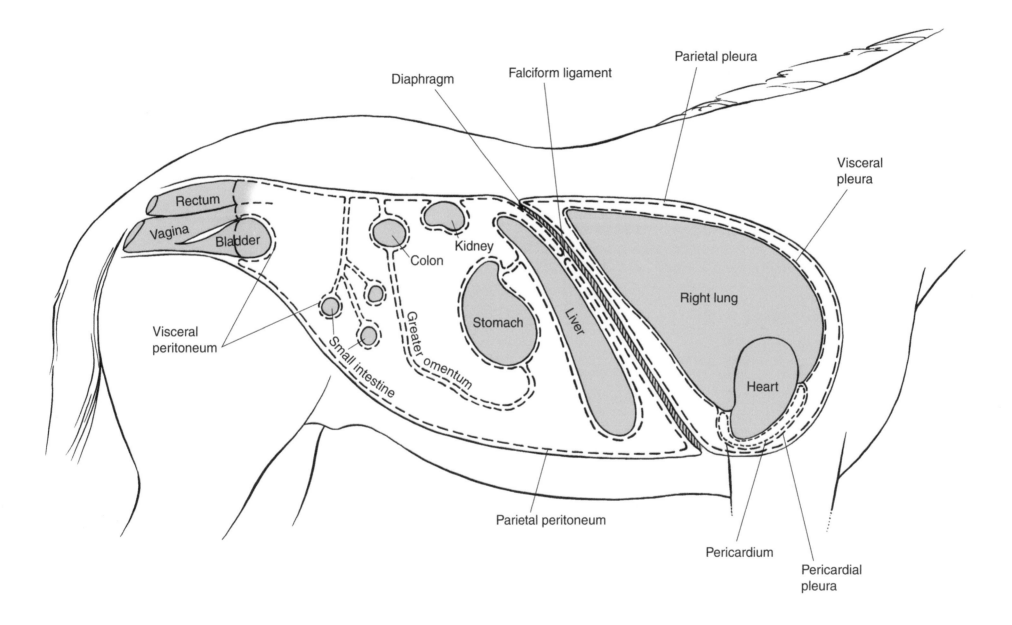

Diaphragm

Falciform ligament

Parietal pleura

Visceral pleura

Rectum

Vagina

Bladder

Colon

Kidney

Right lung

Visceral peritoneum

Stomach

Liver

Heart

Small intestine

Greater omentum

Parietal peritoneum

Pericardium

Pericardial pleura

xix

SECTION 1 THE HORSE (*Equus caballus*)

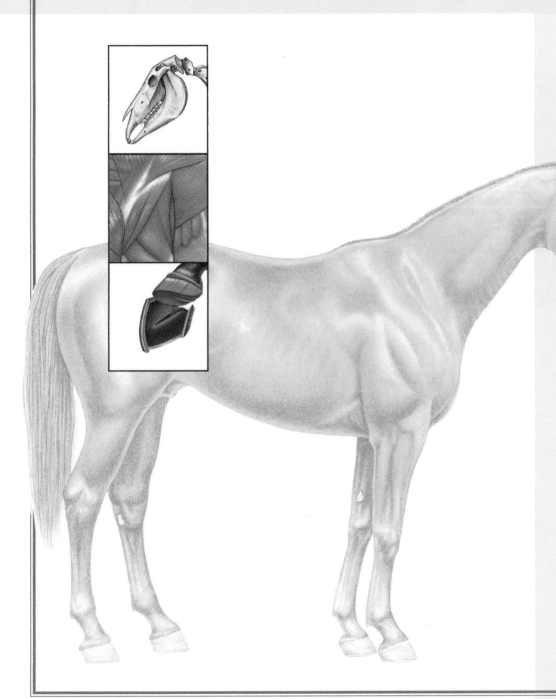

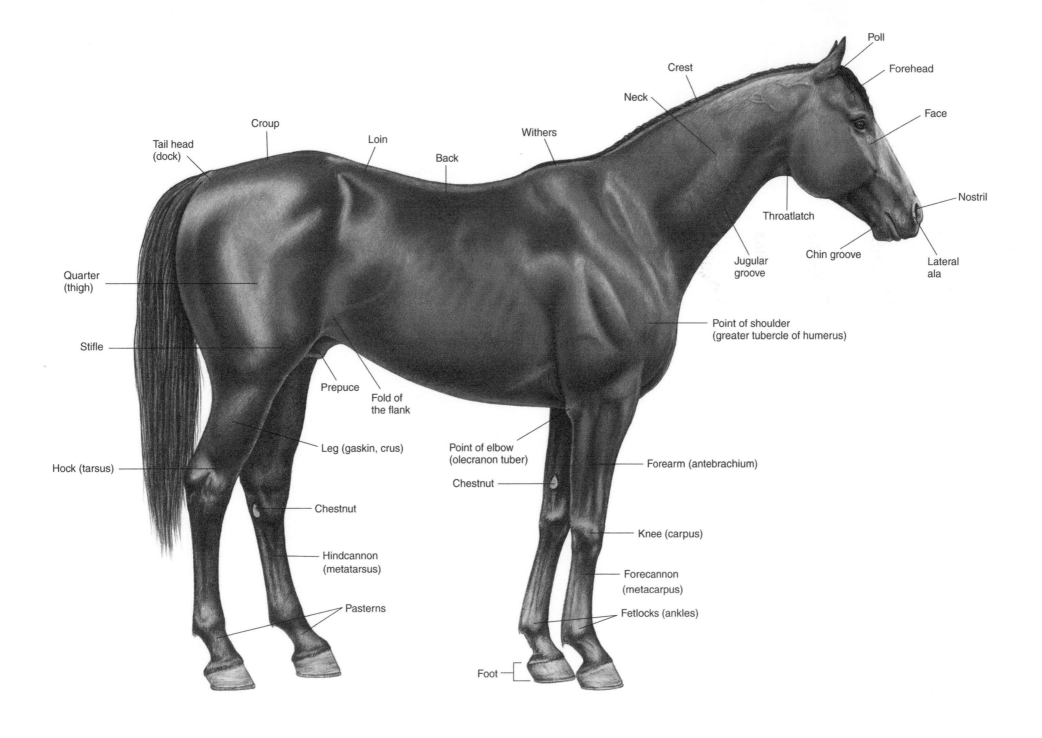

PLATE 1.1 Right lateral view of a stallion.

Poll

Crest

Forehead

Neck

Face

Croup

Loin

Withers

Nostril

Tail head
(dock)

Back

Throatlatch

Chin groove

Lateral
ala

Jugular
groove

Quarter
(thigh)

Point of shoulder
(greater tubercle of humerus)

Stifle

Prepuce

Fold of
the flank

Point of elbow
(olecranon tuber)

Forearm (antebrachium)

Leg (gaskin, crus)

Chestnut

Hock (tarsus)

Knee (carpus)

Chestnut

Forecannon
(metacarpus)

Hindcannon
(metatarsus)

Fetlocks (ankles)

Pasterns

Foot

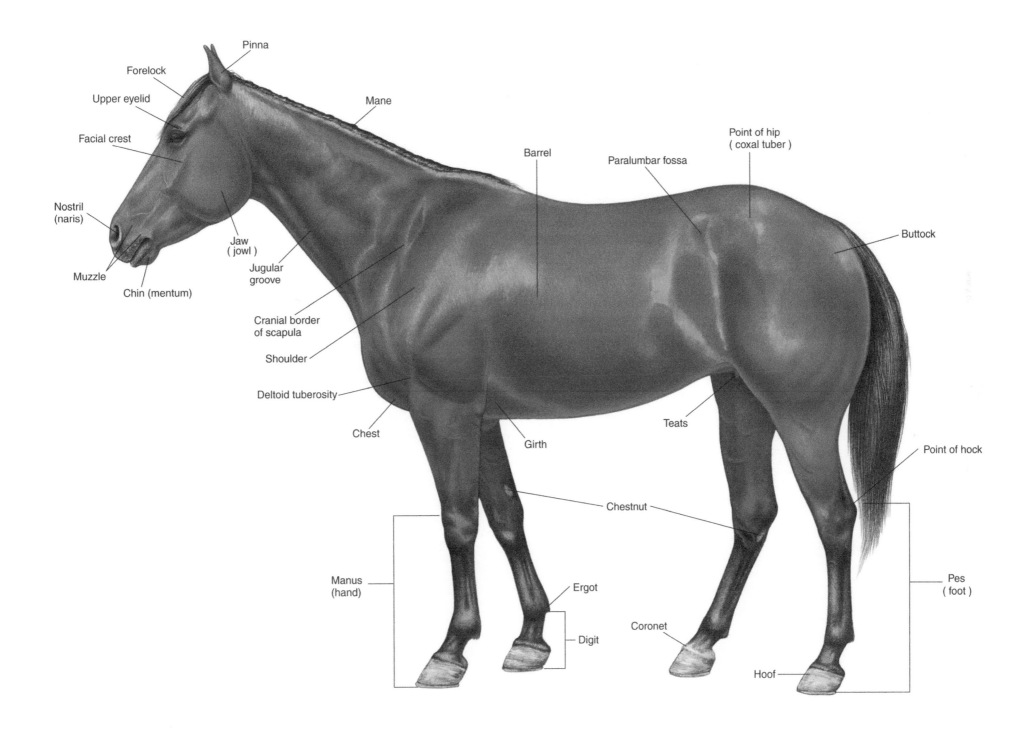

Pinna

Forelock

Upper eyelid

Mane

Point of hip
(coxal tuber)

Facial crest

Barrel

Paralumbar fossa

Nostril
(naris)

Buttock

Jaw
(jowl)

Muzzle

Jugular
groove

Chin (mentum)

Cranial border
of scapula

Shoulder

Deltoid tuberosity

Teats

Chest

Girth

Point of hock

Chestnut

Manus
(hand)

Ergot

Pes
(foot)

Coronet

Digit

Hoof

PLATE 1.2   Left lateral view of a mare.

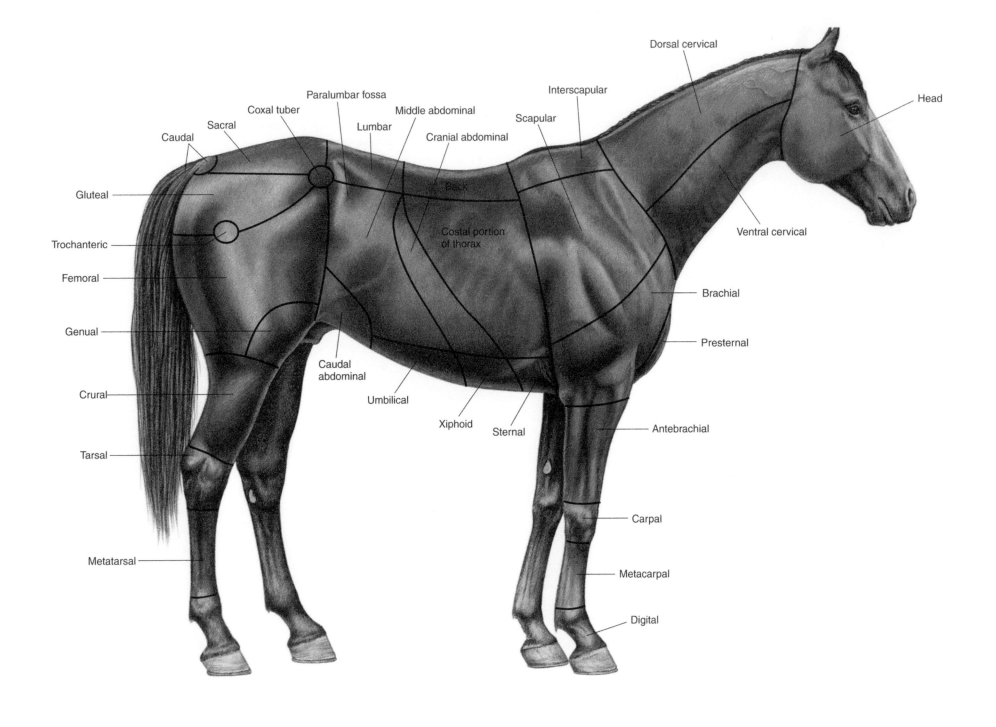

Dorsal cervical

Interscapular

Head

Paralumbar fossa

Coxal tuber

Middle abdominal

Scapular

Sacral

Lumbar

Cranial abdominal

Caudal

Back

Gluteal

Ventral cervical

Costal portion
of thorax

Trochanteric

Femoral

Brachial

Genual

Presternal

Caudal
abdominal

Crural

Umbilical

Antebrachial

Xiphoid

Sternal

Tarsal

Carpal

Metatarsal

Metacarpal

Digital

4

PLATE 1.3   Body regions of the horse. Right lateral view.

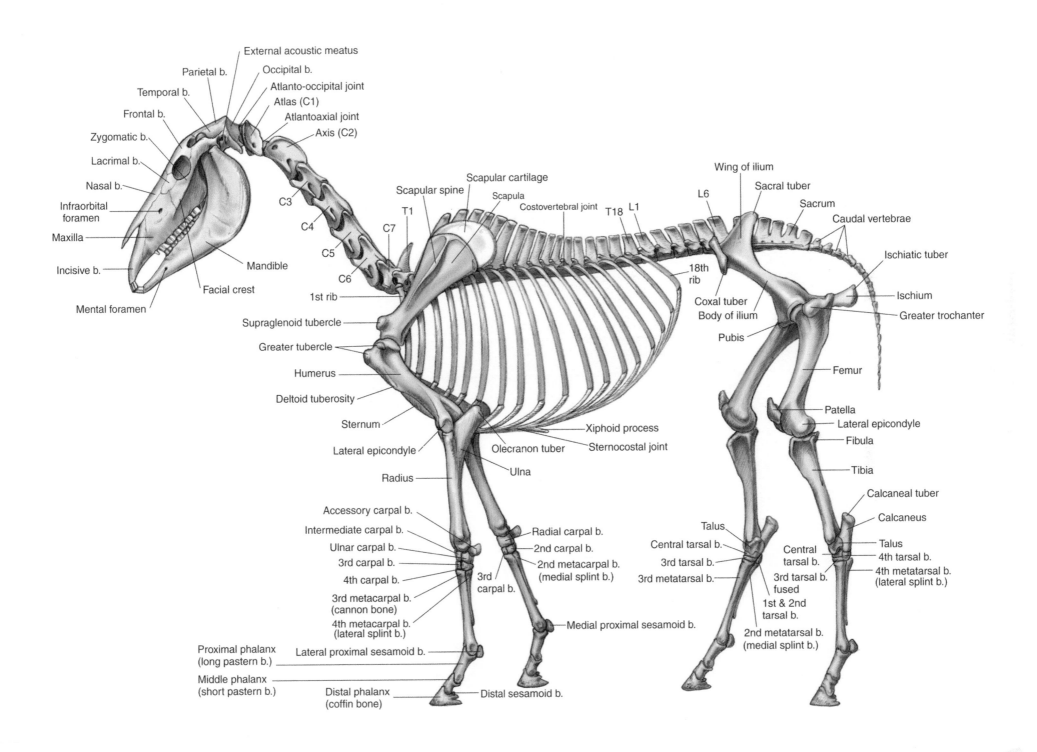

PLATE 1.4   Skeleton of the horse. Left lateral view. C = cervical vertebra,
T = thoracic vertebra, L = lumbar vertebra , b = bone

5

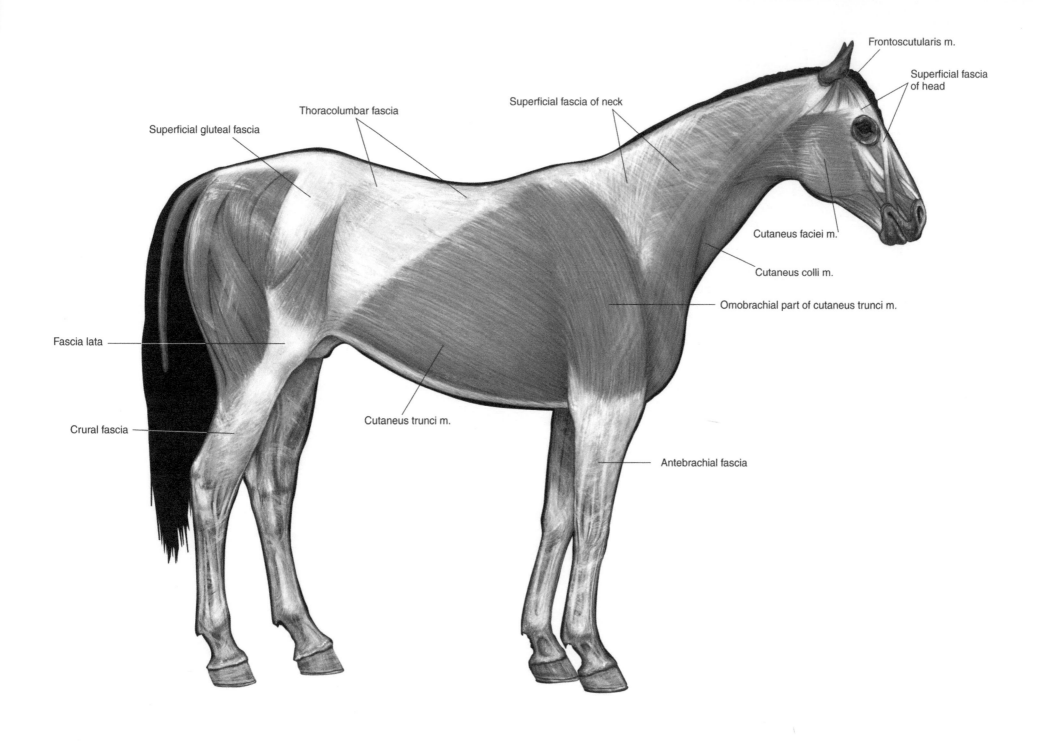

Frontoscutularis m.

Superficial fascia
of head

Superficial fascia of neck

Thoracolumbar fascia

Superficial gluteal fascia

Cutaneus faciei m.

Cutaneus colli m.

Omobrachial part of cutaneus trunci m.

Fascia lata

Cutaneus trunci m.

Crural fascia

Antebrachial fascia

6

PLATE 1.5 Cutaneous muscles and major fasciae of the stallion. Right lateral view. m = muscle

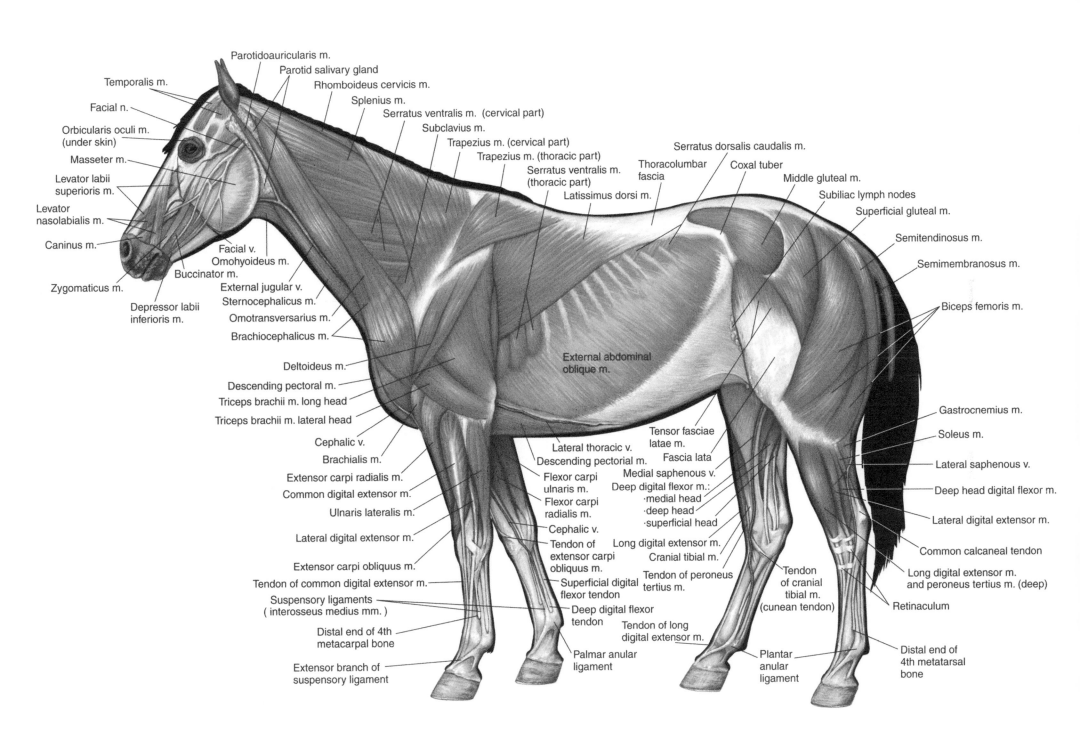

Parotidoauricularis m.
Parotid salivary gland
Rhomboideus cervicis m.
Temporalis m.
Splenius m.
Facial n.
Serratus ventralis m. (cervical part)
Orbicularis oculi m.
(under skin)
Subclavius m.
Masseter m.
Trapezius m. (cervical part)
Levator labii
superioris m.
Trapezius m. (thoracic part)
Serratus dorsalis caudalis m.
Levator
nasolabialis m.
Serratus ventralis m.
(thoracic part)
Thoracolumbar
fascia
Coxal tuber
Middle gluteal m.
Subiliac lymph nodes
Caninus m.
Latissimus dorsi m.
Superficial gluteal m.
Zygomaticus m.
Semitendinosus m.
Facial v.
Omohyoideus m.
Semimembranosus m.
Depressor labii
inferioris m.
Buccinator m.
External jugular v.
Biceps femoris m.
Sternocephalicus m.
Omotransversarius m.
External abdominal
oblique m.
Brachiocephalicus m.
Deltoideus m.
Descending pectoral m.
Triceps brachii m. long head
Gastrocnemius m.
Triceps brachii m. lateral head
Soleus m.
Tensor fasciae
latae m.
Lateral saphenous v.
Cephalic v.
Lateral thoracic v.
Fascia lata
Brachialis m.
Descending pectoral m.
Medial saphenous v.
Deep head digital flexor m.
Extensor carpi radialis m.
Flexor carpi
ulnaris m.
Deep digital flexor m.:
·medial head
·deep head
·superficial head
Lateral digital extensor m.
Common digital extensor m.
Flexor carpi
radialis m.
Ulnaris lateralis m.
Long digital extensor m.
Common calcaneal tendon
Cephalic v.
Lateral digital extensor m.
Cranial tibial m.
Long digital extensor m.
and peroneus tertius m. (deep)
Extensor carpi obliquus m.
Tendon of
extensor carpi
obliquus m.
Tendon of peroneus
tertius m.
Tendon
of cranial
tibial m.
(cunean tendon)
Retinaculum
Tendon of common digital extensor m.
Superficial digital
flexor tendon
Suspensory ligaments
(interosseus medius mm.)
Deep digital flexor
tendon
Distal end
of 4th
metatarsal
bone
Distal end of 4th
metacarpal bone
Tendon of long
digital extensor m.
Plantar
anular
ligament
Extensor branch of
suspensory ligament
Palmar anular
ligament

7

PLATE 1.6 Superficial muscles and veins of the mare. Left lateral view.
m = muscle, n = nerve, v = vein

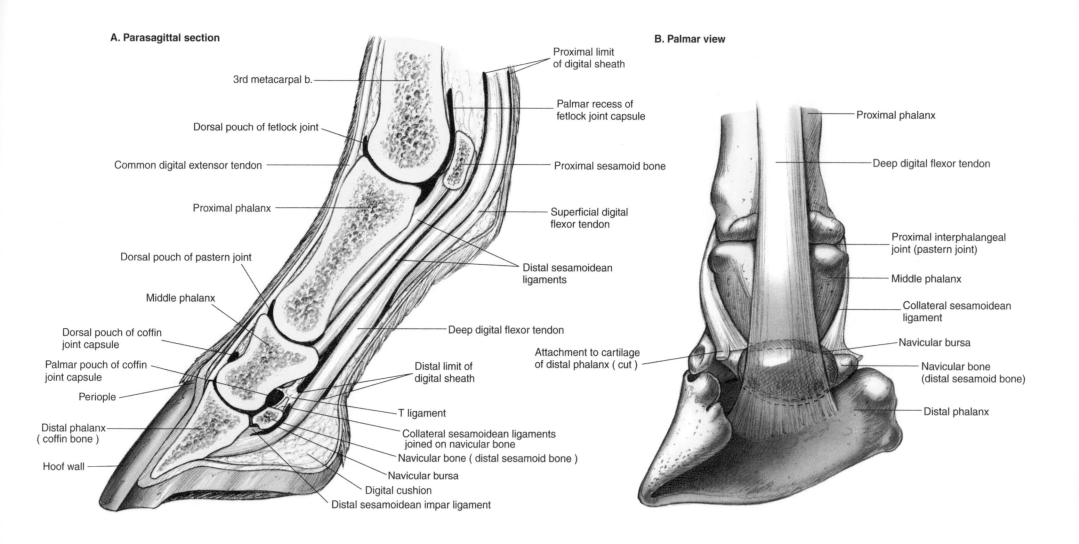

A. Parasagittal section

3rd metacarpal b.

Dorsal pouch of fetlock joint

Common digital extensor tendon

Proximal phalanx

Dorsal pouch of pastern joint

Middle phalanx

Dorsal pouch of coffin
joint capsule

Palmar pouch of coffin
joint capsule

Periople

Distal phalanx
(coffin bone)

Hoof wall

Proximal limit
of digital sheath

Palmar recess of
fetlock joint capsule

Proximal sesamoid bone

Superficial digital
flexor tendon

Distal sesamoidean
ligaments

Deep digital flexor tendon

Distal limit of
digital sheath

T ligament

Collateral sesamoidean ligaments
joined on navicular bone

Navicular bone (distal sesamoid bone)

Navicular bursa

Digital cushion

Distal sesamoidean impar ligament

B. Palmar view

Proximal phalanx

Deep digital flexor tendon

Proximal interphalangeal
joint (pastern joint)

Middle phalanx

Collateral sesamoidean
ligament

Navicular bursa

Navicular bone
(distal sesamoid bone)

Distal phalanx

Attachment to cartilage
of distal phalanx (cut)

PLATE 1.7   A. Parasagittal section of the equine digit. **B.** Palmar (plantar) view of major
structures of the equine digit. Navicular bursa obscures joining of collateral
sesamoidean ligaments on the navicular bone. b = bone

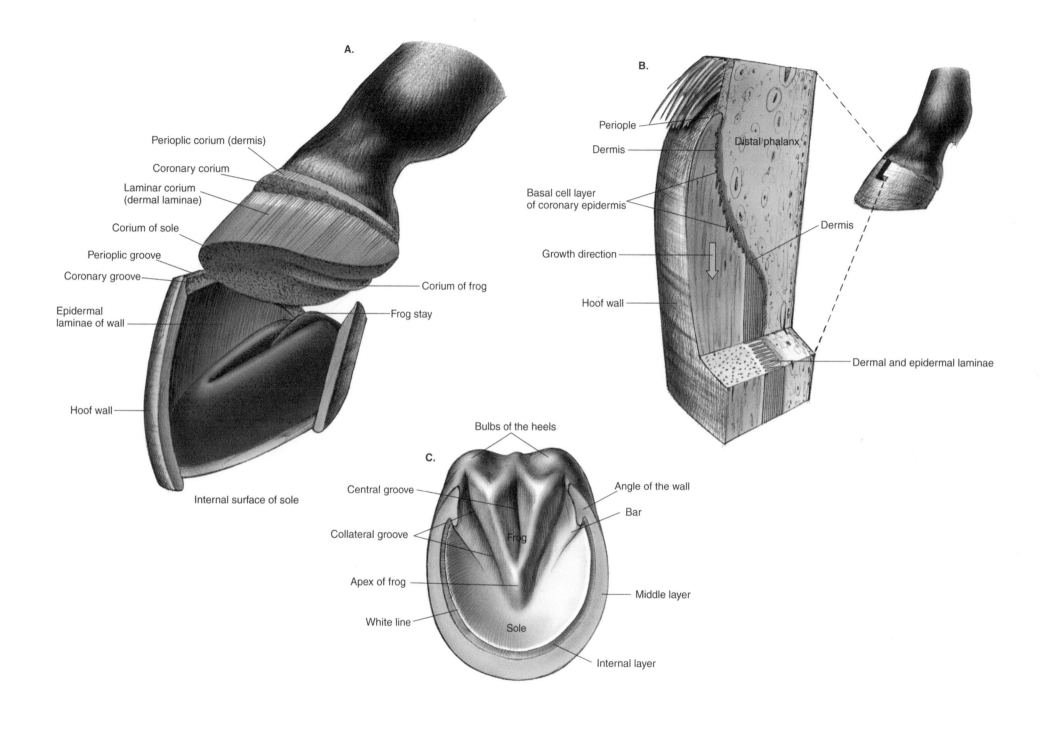

A.

Perioplic corium (dermis)

Coronary corium

Laminar corium
(dermal laminae)

Corium of sole

Perioplic groove

Coronary groove

Epidermal
laminae of wall

Hoof wall

Internal surface of sole

Corium of frog

Frog stay

B.

Periople

Dermis

Basal cell layer
of coronary epidermis

Growth direction

Hoof wall

Distal phalanx

Dermis

Dermal and epidermal laminae

C.

Bulbs of the heels

Central groove

Collateral groove

Apex of frog

White line

Frog

Sole

Angle of the wall

Bar

Middle layer

Internal layer

PLATE 1.8   Relations of the hoof. **A.** Separation of the hoof to show its relations to regions of the
corium. **B.** Three-dimensional dissection to show relations of the hoof wall, coronary
and laminar corium, and distal phalanx. **C.** Solar surface of the hoof.

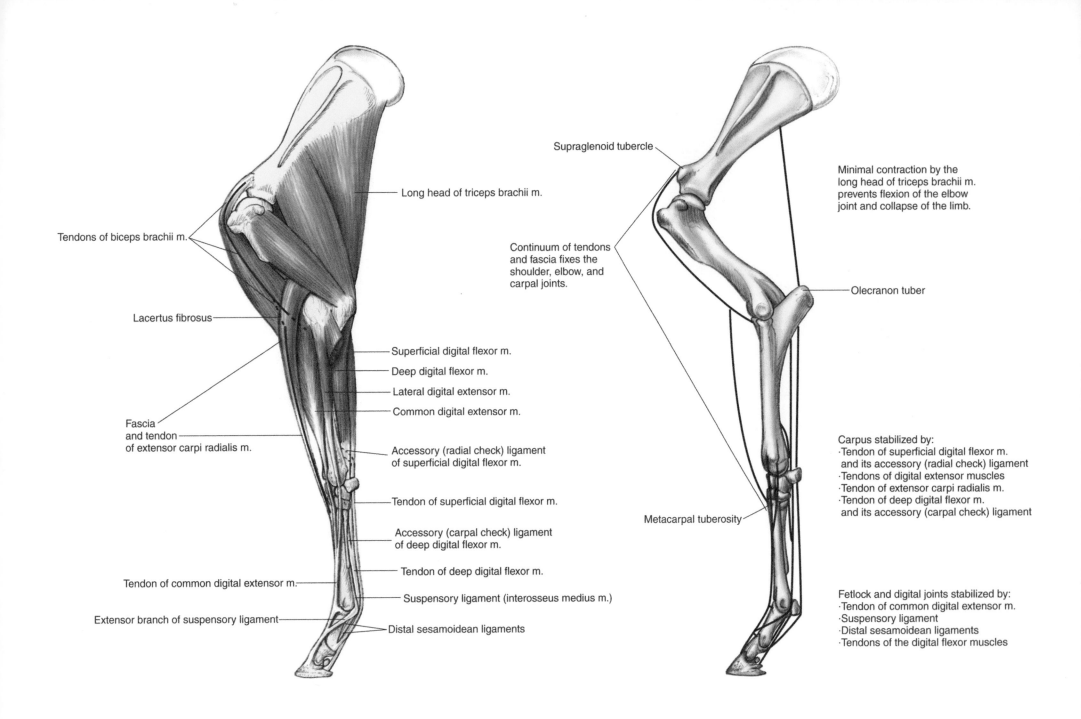

Supraglenoid tubercle

Long head of triceps brachii m.

Tendons of biceps brachii m.

Minimal contraction by the long head of triceps brachii m. prevents flexion of the elbow joint and collapse of the limb.

Continuum of tendons and fascia fixes the shoulder, elbow, and carpal joints.

Lacertus fibrosus

Olecranon tuber

Superficial digital flexor m.

Deep digital flexor m.

Lateral digital extensor m.

Common digital extensor m.

Fascia and tendon of extensor carpi radialis m.

Accessory (radial check) ligament of superficial digital flexor m.

Carpus stabilized by:
·Tendon of superficial digital flexor m. and its accessory (radial check) ligament
·Tendons of digital extensor muscles
·Tendon of extensor carpi radialis m.
·Tendon of deep digital flexor m. and its accessory (carpal check) ligament

Tendon of superficial digital flexor m.

Accessory (carpal check) ligament of deep digital flexor m.

Metacarpal tuberosity

Tendon of deep digital flexor m.

Tendon of common digital extensor m.

Suspensory ligament (interosseus medius m.)

Fetlock and digital joints stabilized by:
·Tendon of common digital extensor m.
·Suspensory ligament
·Distal sesamoidean ligaments
·Tendons of the digital flexor muscles

Extensor branch of suspensory ligament

Distal sesamoidean ligaments

PLATE 1.9   Stay apparatus of the equine forelimb. The continuum of tendons and ligaments with minimal muscular activity stabilizes joints of the forelimb in the standing position. m = muscle

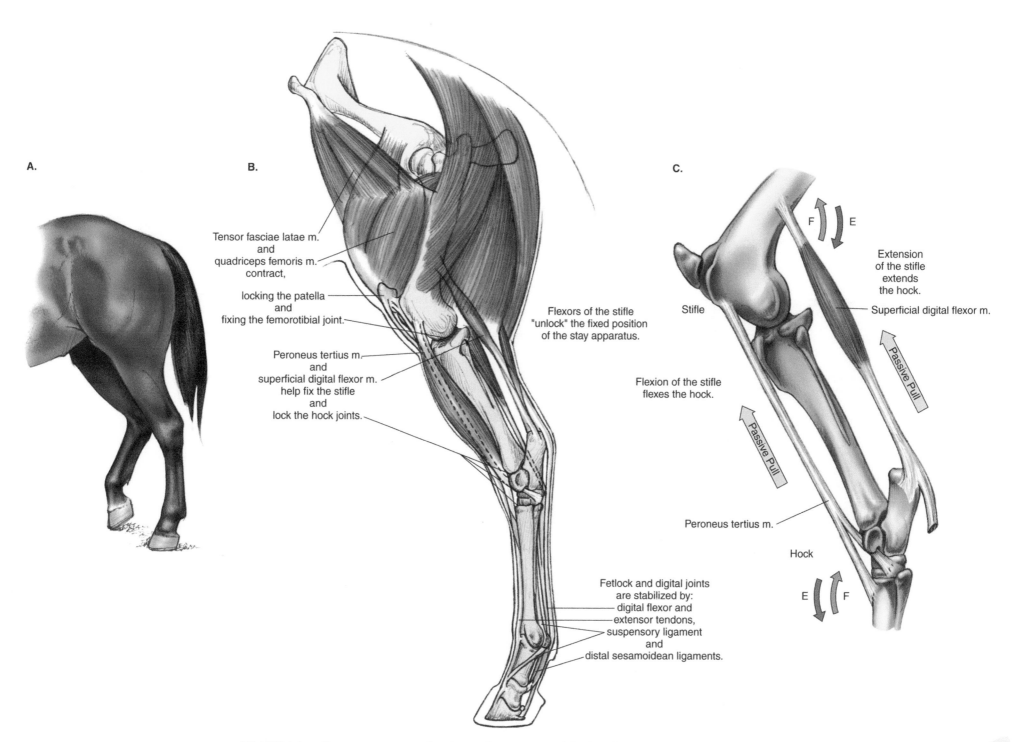

A.

B.

C.

Tensor fasciae latae m.
and
quadriceps femoris m.
contract,

locking the patella
and
fixing the femorotibial joint.

Peroneus tertius m.
and
superficial digital flexor m.
help fix the stifle
and
lock the hock joints.

Flexors of the stifle
"unlock" the fixed position
of the stay apparatus.

Fetlock and digital joints
are stabilized by:
digital flexor and
extensor tendons,
suspensory ligament
and
distal sesamoidean ligaments.

F   E

Extension
of the stifle
extends
the hock.

Stifle

Superficial digital flexor m.

Passive Pull

Flexion of the stifle
flexes the hock.

Passive Pull

Peroneus tertius m.

Hock

E   F

PLATE 1.10 Stay apparatus and reciprocal apparatus of the hindlimb. **A.** One hindlimb partly
flexed with its toe on the ground, and the foot of the opposite limb fixed with minimal
muscular activity by the stay apparatus. **B.** Stay apparatus of the
hindlimb. **C.** The reciprocal apparatus. m = muscle

11

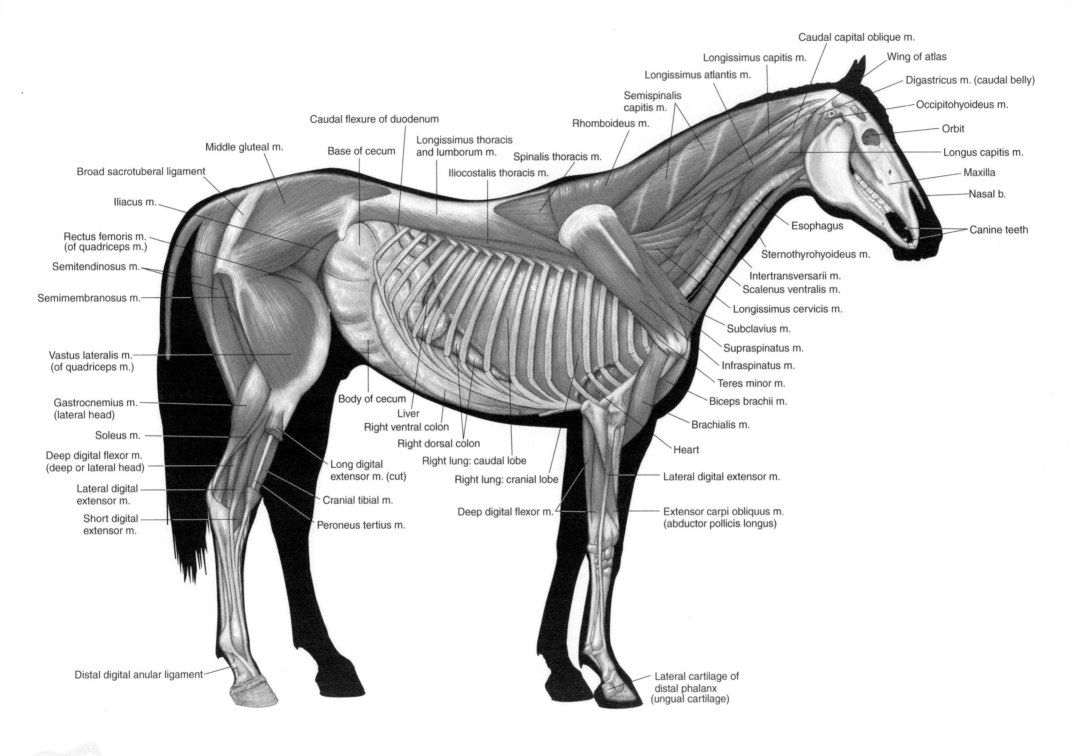

PLATE 1.11 Deep muscles and *in situ* viscera of the stallion.
Right lateral view. m = muscle, b = bone

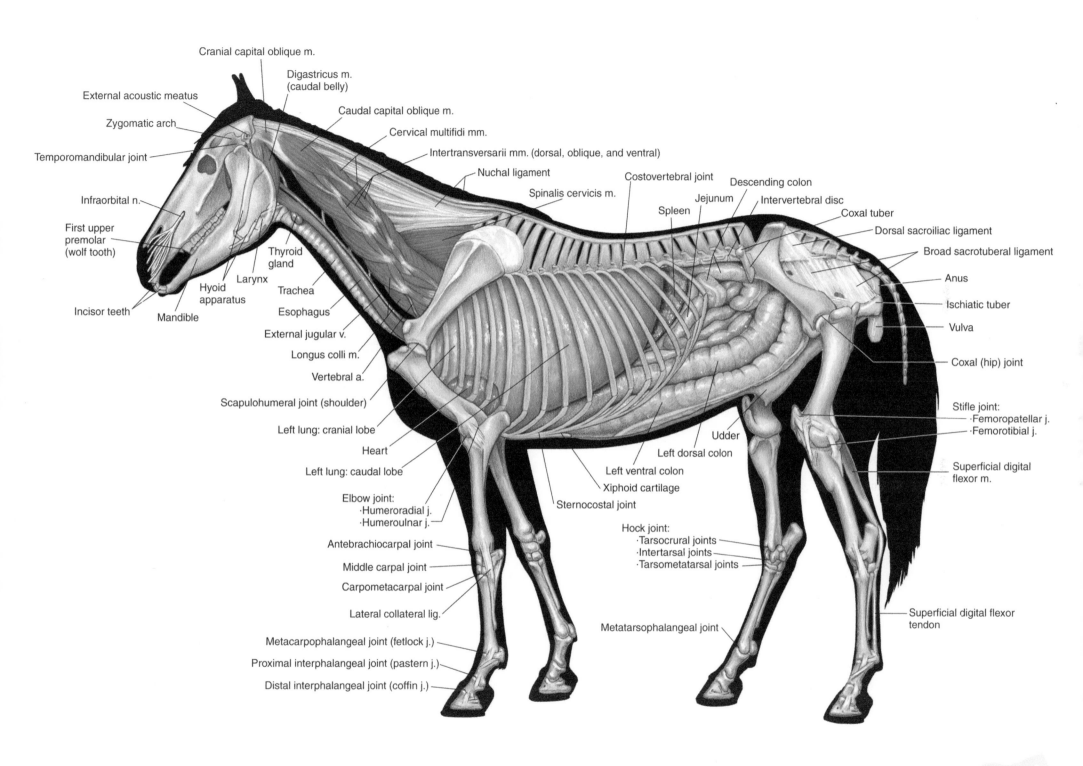

Cranial capital oblique m.

Digastricus m.
(caudal belly)

External acoustic meatus

Caudal capital oblique m.

Zygomatic arch

Cervical multifidi mm.

Temporomandibular joint

Intertransversarii mm. (dorsal, oblique, and ventral)

Nuchal ligament

Costovertebral joint

Descending colon

Infraorbital n.

Spinalis cervicis m.

Jejunum

Intervertebral disc

First upper
premolar
(wolf tooth)

Spleen

Coxal tuber

Dorsal sacroiliac ligament

Broad sacrotuberal ligament

Thyroid
gland

Anus

Larynx

Ischiatic tuber

Incisor teeth

Hyoid
apparatus

Trachea

Vulva

Mandible

Esophagus

External jugular v.

Coxal (hip) joint

Longus colli m.

Vertebral a.

Scapulohumeral joint (shoulder)

Stifle joint:
·Femoropatellar j.
·Femorotibial j.

Left lung: cranial lobe

Udder

Heart

Left dorsal colon

Superficial digital
flexor m.

Left lung: caudal lobe

Left ventral colon

Xiphoid cartilage

Elbow joint:
·Humeroradial j.
·Humeroulnar j.

Sternocostal joint

Hock joint:
·Tarsocrural joints
·Intertarsal joints
·Tarsometatarsal joints

Antebrachiocarpal joint

Middle carpal joint

Carpometacarpal joint

Lateral collateral lig.

Superficial digital flexor
tendon

Metacarpophalangeal joint (fetlock j.)

Metatarsophalangeal joint

Proximal interphalangeal joint (pastern j.)

Distal interphalangeal joint (coffin j.)

13

PLATE 1.12   Deep cervical muscles, major joints, and *in situ* viscera of the mare. Left lateral view.
n = nerve, v = vein, m = muscle, a = artery, j = joint, lig = ligament

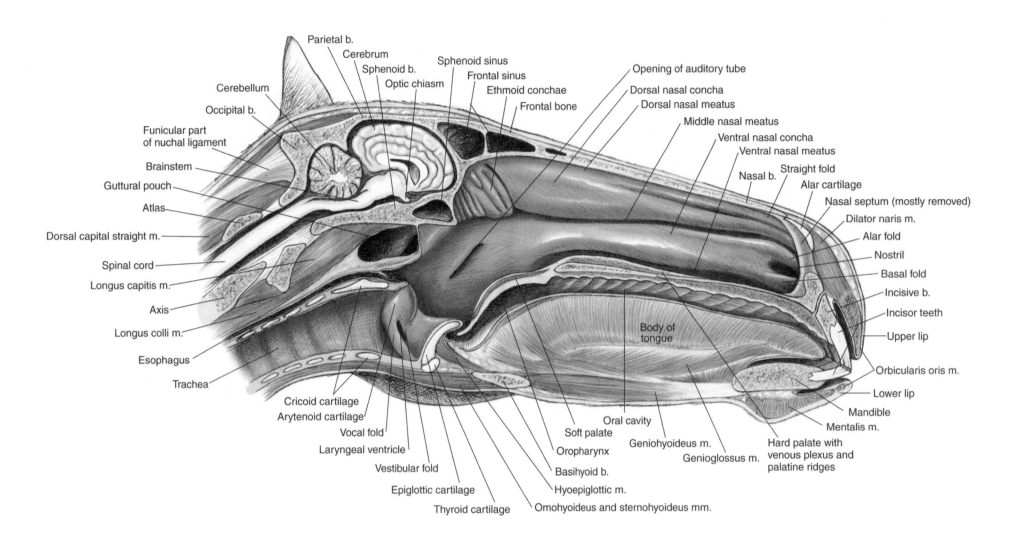

Parietal b.
Cerebrum
Sphenoid b.
Optic chiasm
Sphenoid sinus
Frontal sinus
Ethmoid conchae
Frontal bone
Opening of auditory tube
Dorsal nasal concha
Dorsal nasal meatus
Middle nasal meatus
Ventral nasal concha
Ventral nasal meatus
Nasal b.
Straight fold
Alar cartilage
Nasal septum (mostly removed)
Dilator naris m.
Alar fold
Nostril
Basal fold
Incisive b.
Incisor teeth
Upper lip
Orbicularis oris m.
Lower lip
Mandible
Mentalis m.
Hard palate with venous plexus and palatine ridges
Genioglossus m.
Geniohyoideus m.
Oral cavity
Body of tongue
Soft palate
Oropharynx
Basihyoid b.
Hyoepiglottic m.
Omohyoideus and sternohyoideus mm.
Thyroid cartilage
Epiglottic cartilage
Vestibular fold
Laryngeal ventricle
Vocal fold
Arytenoid cartilage
Cricoid cartilage
Trachea
Esophagus
Longus colli m.
Axis
Longus capitis m.
Spinal cord
Dorsal capital straight m.
Atlas
Guttural pouch
Brainstem
Funicular part of nuchal ligament
Occipital b.
Cerebellum

PLATE 1.13 Median section of the horse's head. Nasal septum mostly removed.
b = bone, m = muscle

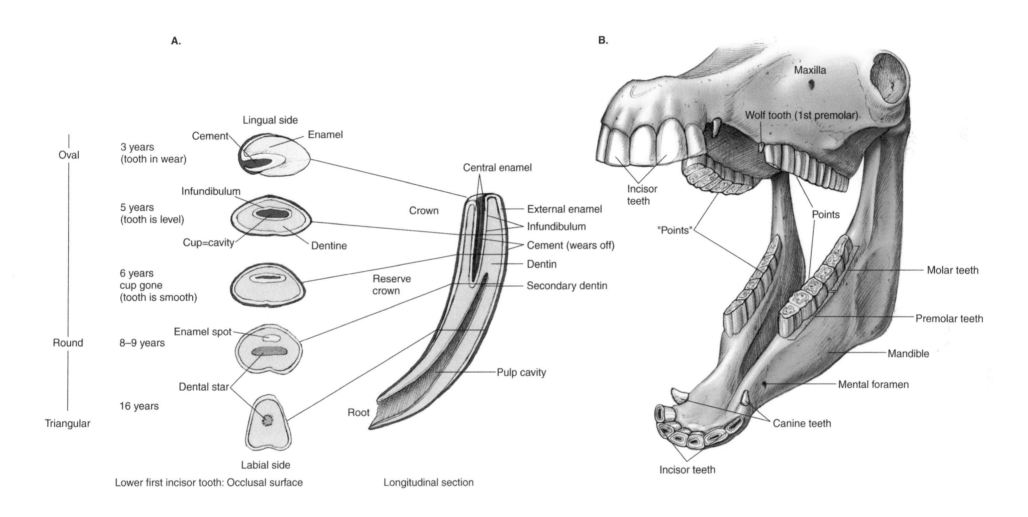

A.

Oval

Round

Triangular

Lingual side

Cement   Enamel

3 years
(tooth in wear)

Infundibulum

5 years
(tooth is level)

Cup=cavity   Dentine

6 years
cup gone
(tooth is smooth)

Enamel spot

8–9 years

Dental star

16 years

Labial side

Lower first incisor tooth: Occlusal surface

Central enamel

Crown

External enamel

Infundibulum

Cement (wears off)

Dentin

Reserve
crown

Secondary dentin

Pulp cavity

Root

Longitudinal section

B.

Maxilla

Wolf tooth (1st premolar)

Incisor
teeth

"Points"

Points

Molar teeth

Premolar teeth

Mandible

Mental foramen

Canine teeth

Incisor teeth

PLATE 1.14   **A.** Occlusal (grinding) surfaces of an equine lower first incisor tooth related to continuous eruption and wear. Approximate levels at advancing ages indicated on a longitudinal section. **B.** Complete dentition of the male horse circa 5 years of age.

15

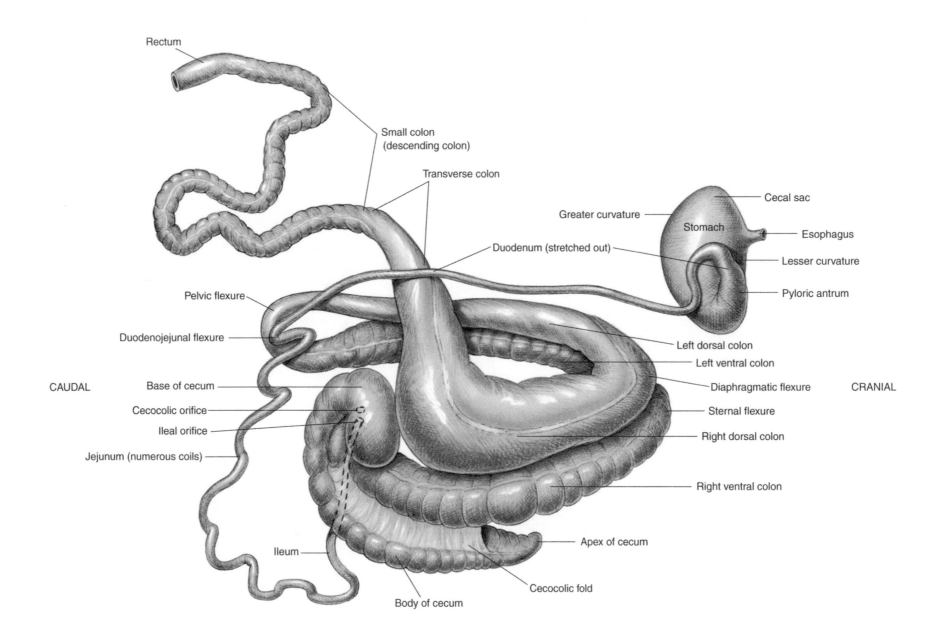

Rectum

Small colon
(descending colon)

Transverse colon

Cecal sac

Greater curvature

Stomach

Esophagus

Duodenum (stretched out)

Lesser curvature

Pyloric antrum

Pelvic flexure

Duodenojejunal flexure

Left dorsal colon

Left ventral colon

Diaphragmatic flexure

CAUDAL

Base of cecum

Cecocolic orifice

Ileal orifice

Jejunum (numerous coils)

CRANIAL

Sternal flexure

Right dorsal colon

Right ventral colon

Apex of cecum

Ileum

Cecocolic fold

Body of cecum

16

PLATE 1.15 Isolated stomach and intestines of the horse.

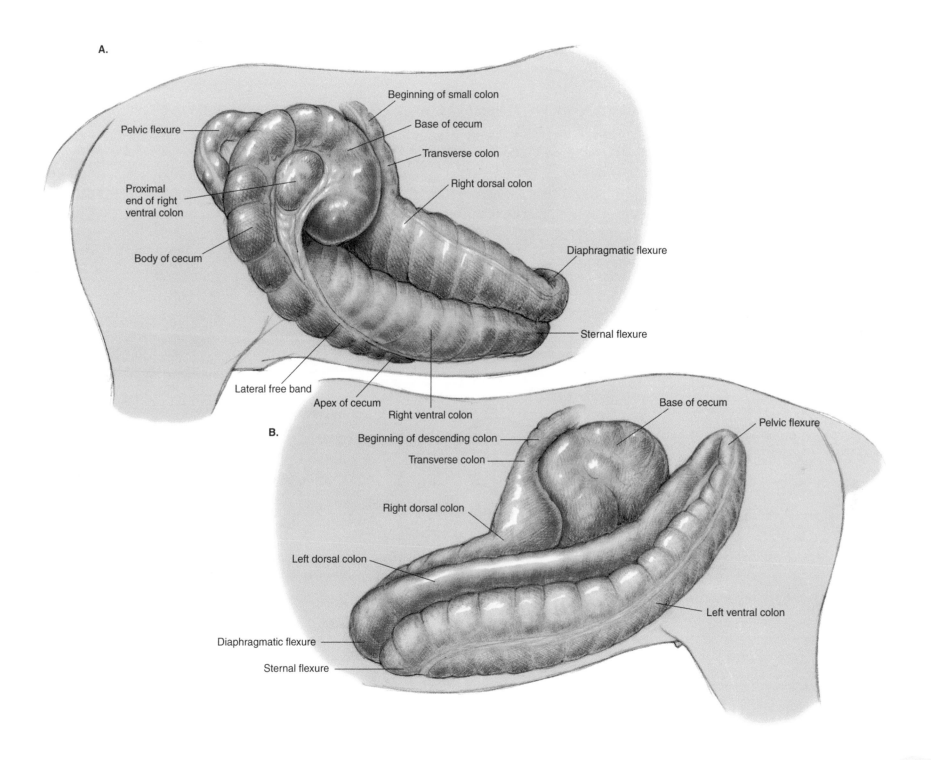

A.

Pelvic flexure

Proximal
end of right
ventral colon

Body of cecum

Beginning of small colon

Base of cecum

Transverse colon

Right dorsal colon

Diaphragmatic flexure

Sternal flexure

Lateral free band

Apex of cecum

Right ventral colon

B.

Beginning of descending colon

Transverse colon

Right dorsal colon

Left dorsal colon

Base of cecum

Pelvic flexure

Left ventral colon

Diaphragmatic flexure

Sternal flexure

PLATE 1.16   Equine cecum, large (ascending) colon, and transverse colon *in situ*.
A. Right lateral view. **B.** Left lateral view.

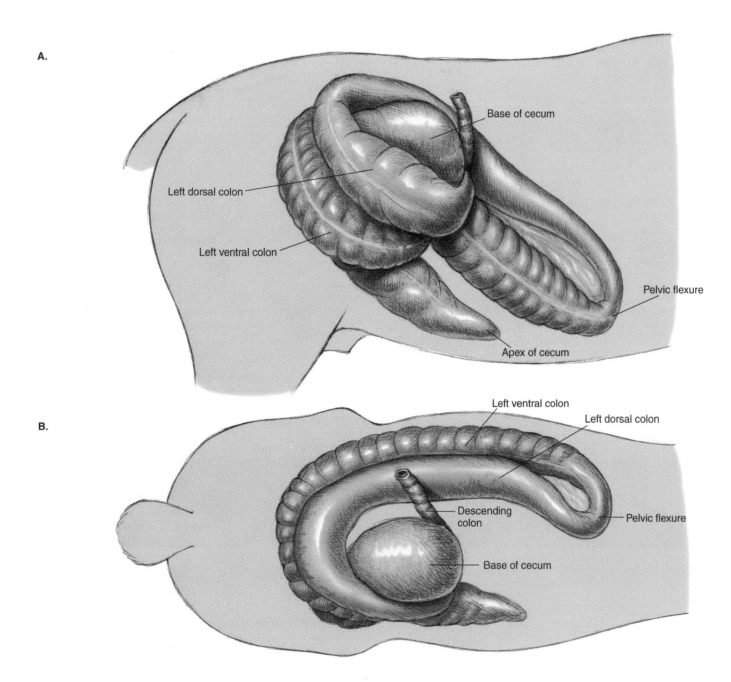

A.

Base of cecum

Left dorsal colon

Left ventral colon

Pelvic flexure

Apex of cecum

B.

Left ventral colon

Left dorsal colon

Descending colon

Pelvic flexure

Base of cecum

PLATE 1.17   Clinical condition: Right dorsal displacement of the large colon. **A.** Right lateral view.
B. Dorsal view. This displacement is a common cause of colic in adult horses. Most commonly, the
large colon moves from the left side of the abdomen, courses caudad between the right body wall
and the cecum, and comes to lie again in the left portion of the abdomen with the pelvic flexure
facing toward the diaphragm. In many cases, the pelvic flexure will not migrate that far
craniad and will instead be located in the caudal aspect of the abdomen on either
side of the body or the median plane.

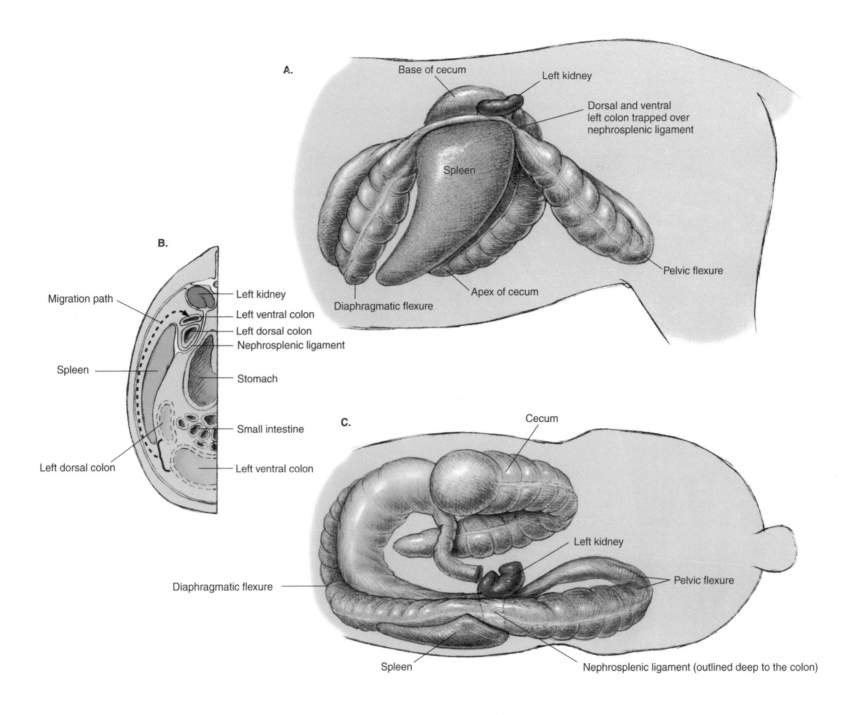

PLATE 1.18   Clinical condition: Left dorsal displacement of the large colon. **A.** Left lateral view.
B. Cross-section of the left side of the abdomen. Caudocranial view. **C.** Dorsal view. In this
displacement, the left colon moves dorsad and becomes entrapped over the nephrosplenic
ligament. The abnormal position of the left colon can often be confirmed by rectal
examination, and, many times, left dorsal displacement can be corrected by
anesthetizing and rolling the horse to free the entrapment.

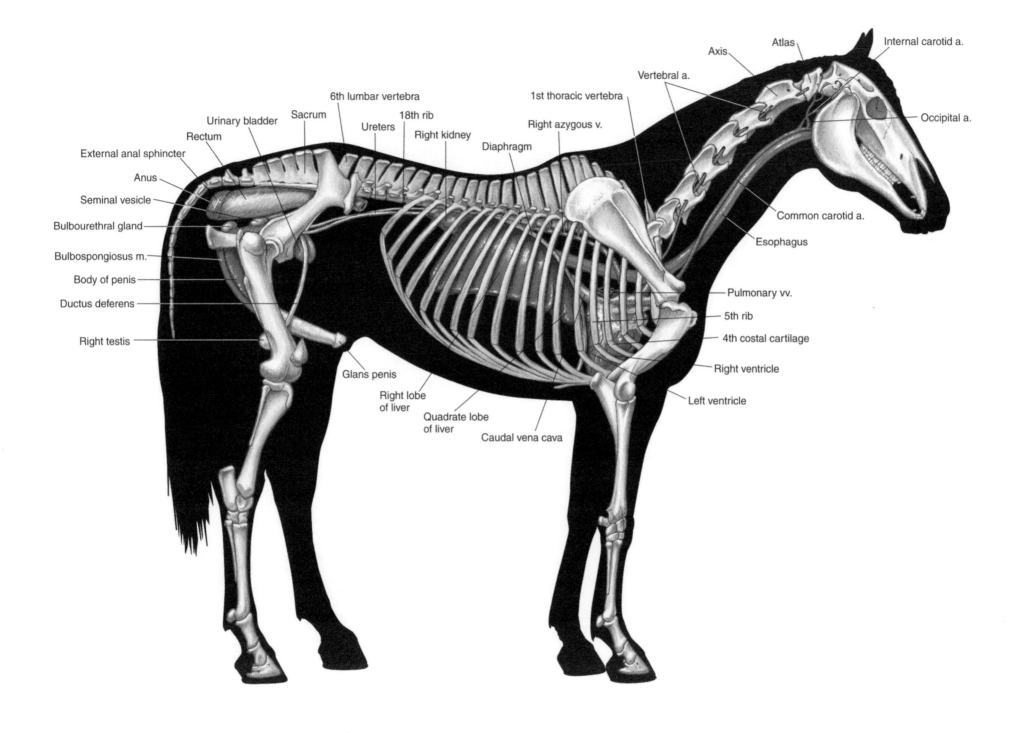

External anal sphincter

Rectum

Urinary bladder

Sacrum

6th lumbar vertebra

Ureters

18th rib

Right kidney

Diaphragm

Right azygous v.

1st thoracic vertebra

Vertebral a.

Axis

Atlas

Internal carotid a.

Anus

Seminal vesicle

Bulbourethral gland

Bulbospongiosus m.

Body of penis

Ductus deferens

Right testis

Glans penis

Right lobe of liver

Quadrate lobe of liver

Caudal vena cava

Occipital a.

Common carotid a.

Esophagus

Pulmonary vv.

5th rib

4th costal cartilage

Right ventricle

Left ventricle

20

PLATE 1.19 Reproductive organs, urinary organs, liver, heart, and adjacent major vessels related to the skeleton of the stallion. Intestines and lungs are removed. Right lateral view. v = vein, a = artery, m = muscle

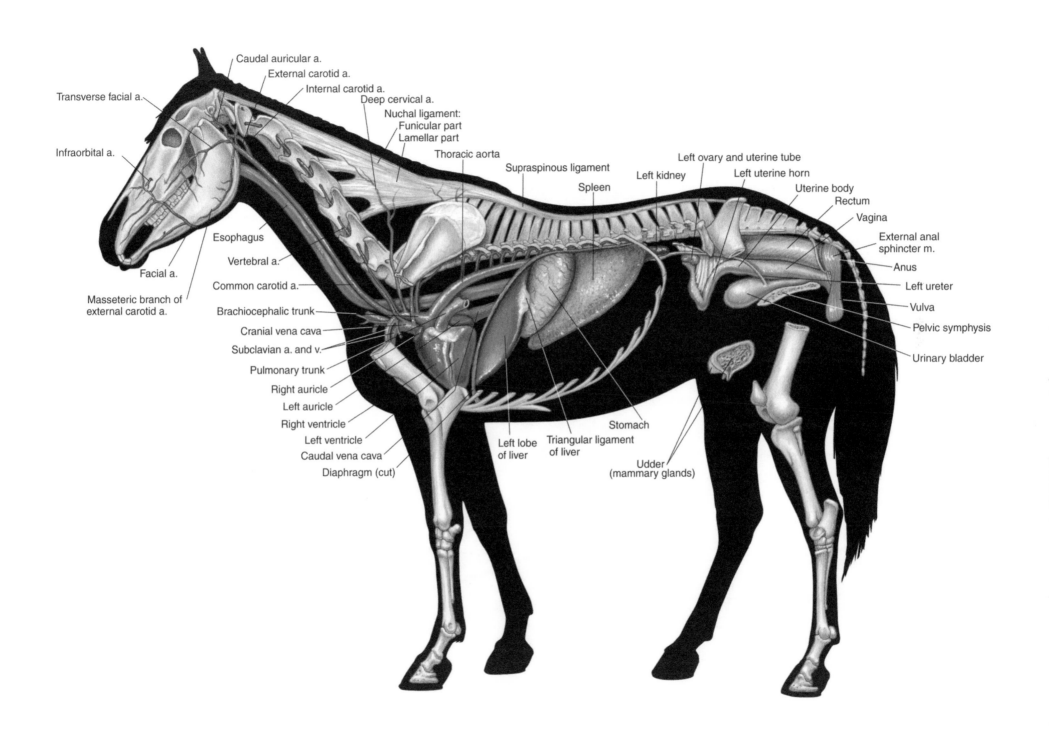

Caudal auricular a.
External carotid a.
Internal carotid a.
Deep cervical a.
Nuchal ligament:
Funicular part
Lamellar part
Thoracic aorta
Transverse facial a.
Infraorbital a.
Facial a.
Masseteric branch of external carotid a.
Esophagus
Vertebral a.
Common carotid a.
Brachiocephalic trunk
Cranial vena cava
Subclavian a. and v.
Pulmonary trunk
Right auricle
Left auricle
Right ventricle
Left ventricle
Caudal vena cava
Diaphragm (cut)
Left lobe of liver
Triangular ligament of liver
Stomach
Udder (mammary glands)
Supraspinous ligament
Spleen
Left kidney
Left ovary and uterine tube
Left uterine horn
Uterine body
Rectum
Vagina
External anal sphincter m.
Anus
Left ureter
Vulva
Pelvic symphysis
Urinary bladder

PLATE 1.20   Heart and some adjacent major vessels, abdominal and pelvic viscera, and udder (mammary glands) of the mare. Intestines and lungs are removed. Left lateral view. a = artery, v = vein, m = muscle

21

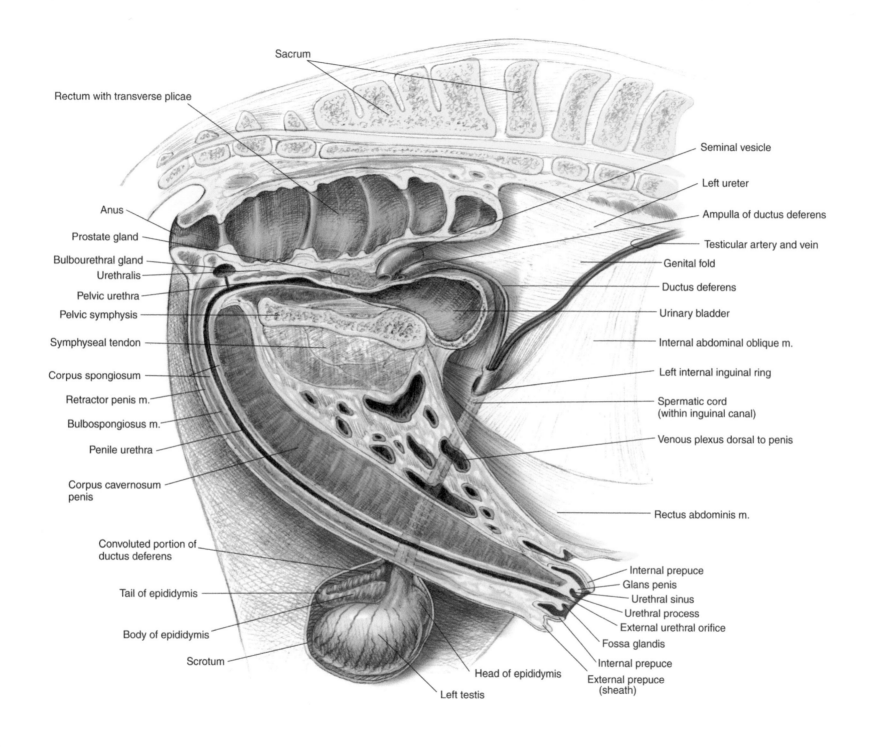

Sacrum

Rectum with transverse plicae

Seminal vesicle

Left ureter

Ampulla of ductus deferens

Anus

Testicular artery and vein

Prostate gland

Genital fold

Bulbourethral gland

Ductus deferens

Urethralis

Pelvic urethra

Urinary bladder

Pelvic symphysis

Symphyseal tendon

Internal abdominal oblique m.

Corpus spongiosum

Left internal inguinal ring

Retractor penis m.

Spermatic cord
(within inguinal canal)

Bulbospongiosus m.

Venous plexus dorsal to penis

Penile urethra

Corpus cavernosum
penis

Rectus abdominis m.

Convoluted portion of
ductus deferens

Internal prepuce
Glans penis

Tail of epididymis

Urethral sinus
Urethral process

Body of epididymis

External urethral orifice

Fossa glandis

Scrotum

Internal prepuce

Head of epididymis

External prepuce
(sheath)

Left testis

22

PLATE 1.21   Relations of the reproductive organs of the stallion.
Median section, right lateral view. m = muscle

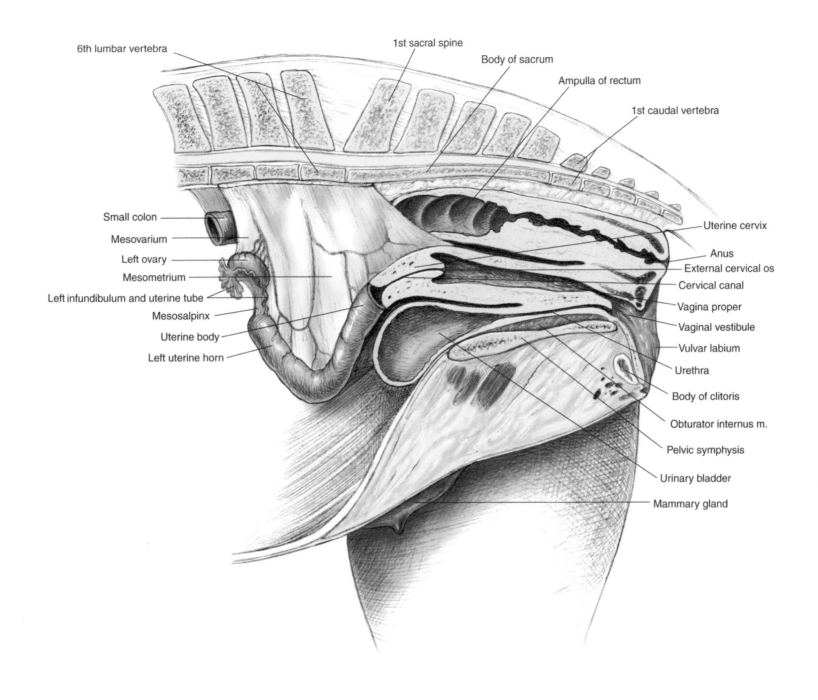

6th lumbar vertebra

1st sacral spine

Body of sacrum

Ampulla of rectum

1st caudal vertebra

Small colon

Mesovarium

Left ovary

Mesometrium

Left infundibulum and uterine tube

Mesosalpinx

Uterine body

Left uterine horn

Uterine cervix

Anus

External cervical os

Cervical canal

Vagina proper

Vaginal vestibule

Vulvar labium

Urethra

Body of clitoris

Obturator internus m.

Pelvic symphysis

Urinary bladder

Mammary gland

23

PLATE 1.22 Relations of the reproductive organs of the mare. Partial median section.
Left lateral view. m = muscle

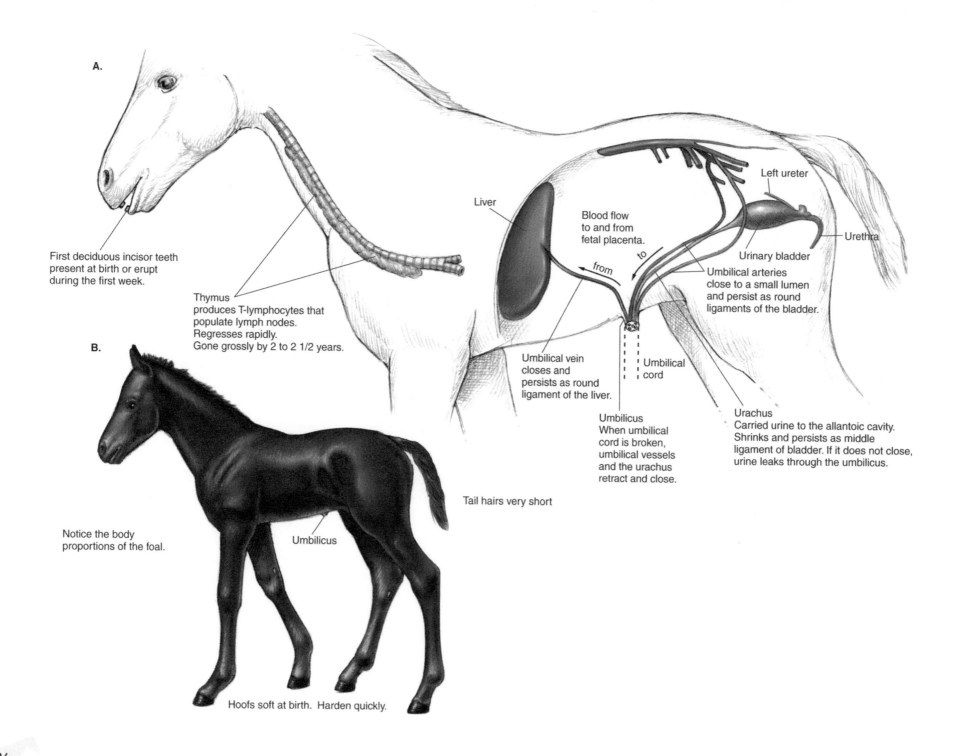

A.

First deciduous incisor teeth present at birth or erupt during the first week.

Thymus
produces T-lymphocytes that populate lymph nodes. Regresses rapidly. Gone grossly by 2 to 2 1/2 years.

Liver

Blood flow to and from fetal placenta.

from

to

Left ureter

Urethra

Urinary bladder

Umbilical arteries close to a small lumen and persist as round ligaments of the bladder.

Umbilical vein closes and persists as round ligament of the liver.

Umbilical cord

Umbilicus
When umbilical cord is broken, umbilical vessels and the urachus retract and close.

Urachus
Carried urine to the allantoic cavity. Shrinks and persists as middle ligament of bladder. If it does not close, urine leaks through the umbilicus.

Tail hairs very short

B.

Notice the body proportions of the foal.

Umbilicus

Hoofs soft at birth. Harden quickly.

24

PLATE 1.23 Neonatal organs of the foal. Left lateral view.

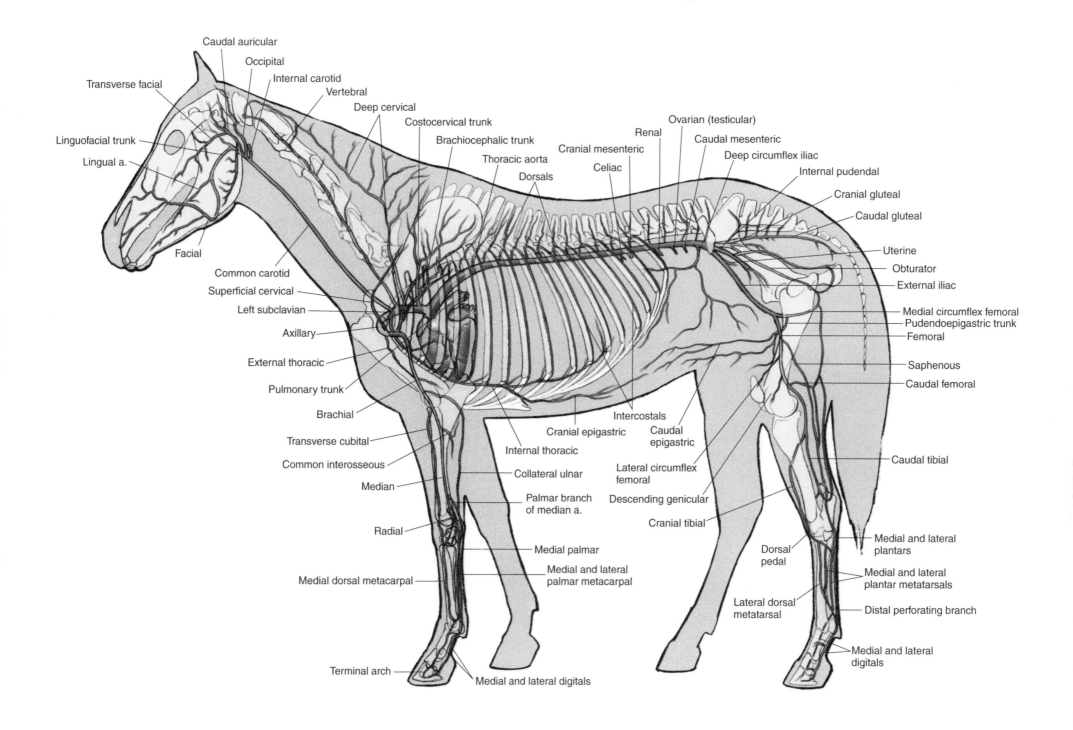

Caudal auricular
Occipital
Internal carotid
Vertebral
Deep cervical
Costocervical trunk
Brachiocephalic trunk
Thoracic aorta
Dorsals
Cranial mesenteric
Celiac
Renal
Ovarian (testicular)
Caudal mesenteric
Deep circumflex iliac
Internal pudendal
Cranial gluteal
Caudal gluteal
Uterine
Obturator
External iliac
Medial circumflex femoral
Pudendoepigastric trunk
Femoral
Saphenous
Caudal femoral
Caudal tibial
Descending genicular
Cranial tibial
Dorsal pedal
Lateral dorsal metatarsal
Medial and lateral plantars
Medial and lateral plantar metatarsals
Distal perforating branch
Medial and lateral digitals

Transverse facial
Linguofacial trunk
Lingual a.
Facial
Common carotid
Superficial cervical
Left subclavian
Axillary
External thoracic
Pulmonary trunk
Brachial
Transverse cubital
Common interosseous
Median
Radial
Terminal arch
Medial dorsal metacarpal
Medial and lateral palmar metacarpal
Medial palmar
Palmar branch of median a.
Collateral ulnar
Internal thoracic
Cranial epigastric
Intercostals
Caudal epigastric
Lateral circumflex femoral
Medial and lateral digitals

25

PLATE 1.24 Major arteries of the mare. Left lateral view. a = artery

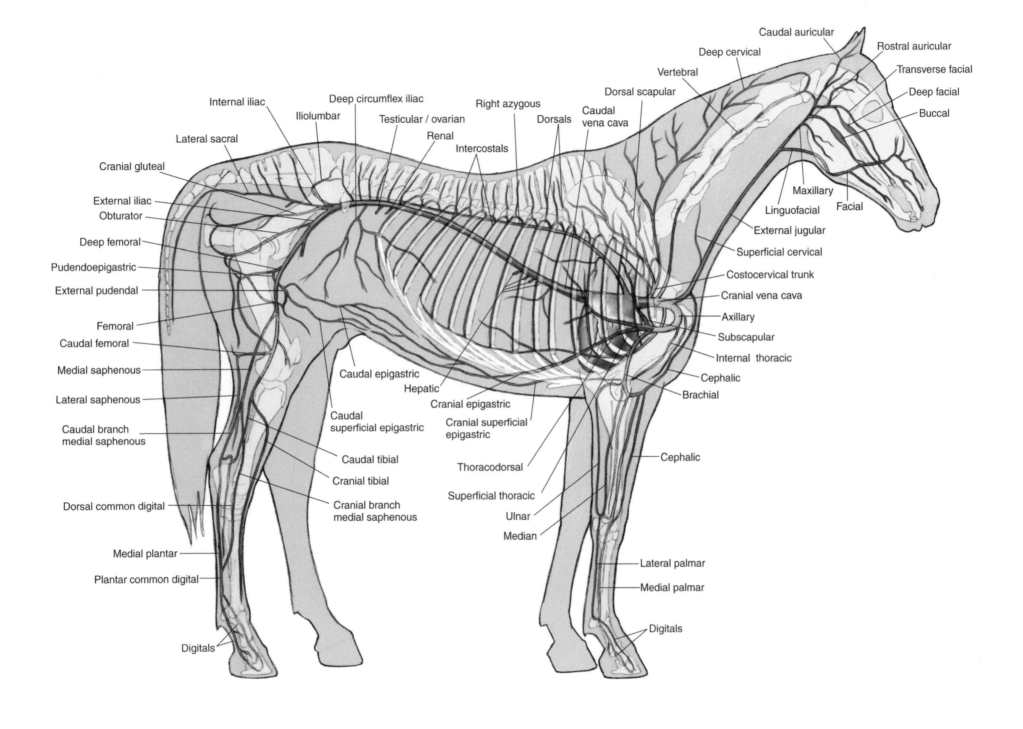

Caudal auricular
Rostral auricular
Deep cervical
Transverse facial
Vertebral
Deep facial
Dorsal scapular
Buccal
Internal iliac
Deep circumflex iliac
Right azygous
Caudal
vena cava
Iliolumbar
Testicular / ovarian
Dorsals
Lateral sacral
Renal
Intercostals
Cranial gluteal
Maxillary
External iliac
Linguofacial
Facial
Obturator
External jugular
Deep femoral
Superficial cervical
Pudendoepigastric
Costocervical trunk
External pudendal
Cranial vena cava
Axillary
Femoral
Subscapular
Caudal femoral
Internal thoracic
Medial saphenous
Caudal epigastric
Cephalic
Lateral saphenous
Hepatic
Brachial
Cranial epigastric
Caudal branch
medial saphenous
Caudal
superficial epigastric
Cranial superficial
epigastric
Cephalic
Caudal tibial
Thoracodorsal
Cranial tibial
Superficial thoracic
Dorsal common digital
Cranial branch
medial saphenous
Ulnar
Median
Lateral palmar
Medial plantar
Medial palmar
Plantar common digital
Digitals
Digitals

26

PLATE 1.25   Major veins of the stallion. Portal system excluded. Right lateral view.

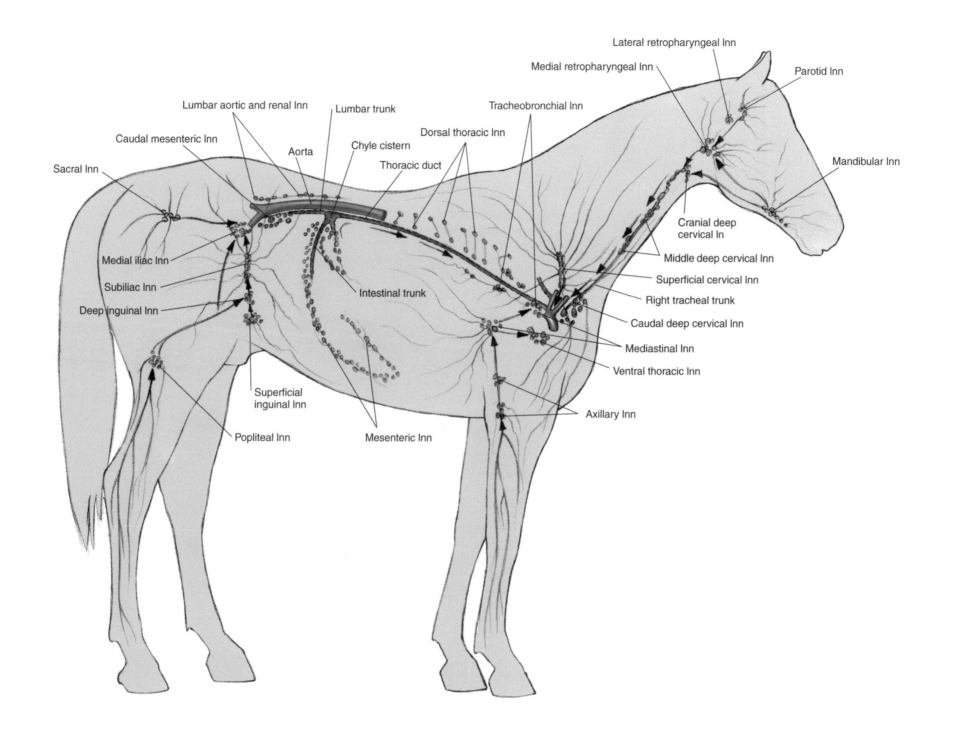

Lateral retropharyngeal lnn

Medial retropharyngeal lnn

Parotid lnn

Lumbar aortic and renal lnn

Lumbar trunk

Tracheobronchial lnn

Caudal mesenteric lnn

Aorta

Chyle cistern

Dorsal thoracic lnn

Mandibular lnn

Sacral lnn

Thoracic duct

Cranial deep cervical ln

Medial iliac lnn

Middle deep cervical lnn

Subiliac lnn

Intestinal trunk

Superficial cervical lnn

Deep inguinal lnn

Right tracheal trunk

Caudal deep cervical lnn

Mediastinal lnn

Superficial inguinal lnn

Ventral thoracic lnn

Popliteal lnn

Mesenteric lnn

Axillary lnn

PLATE 1.26 Lymph nodes and vessels of the horse. Right lateral view. *Arrows* indicate the flow of lymph. Lymph node groups in the horse consist of up to dozens of lymph nodes ranging in size from a few millimeters to 2 centimeters in diameter. ln = lymph node

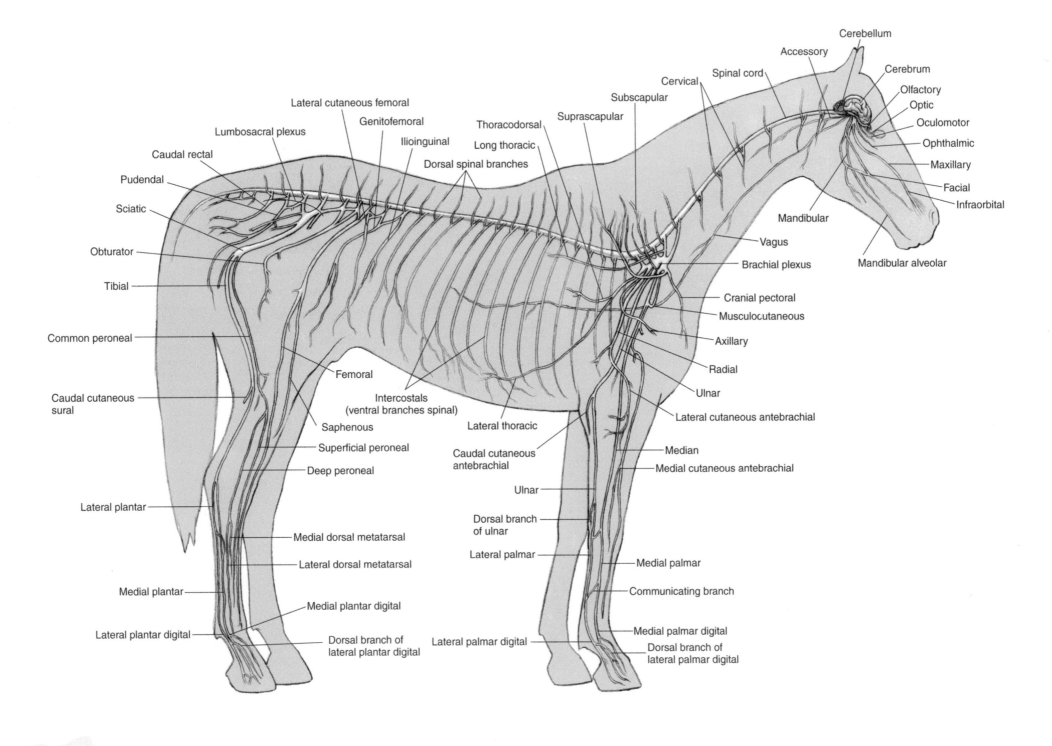

Cerebellum

Accessory

Cervical

Spinal cord

Cerebrum

Olfactory

Optic

Oculomotor

Ophthalmic

Subscapular

Suprascapular

Thoracodorsal

Lateral cutaneous femoral

Genitofemoral

Ilioinguinal

Long thoracic

Dorsal spinal branches

Maxillary

Lumbosacral plexus

Facial

Caudal rectal

Infraorbital

Pudendal

Mandibular

Sciatic

Mandibular alveolar

Vagus

Obturator

Brachial plexus

Tibial

Cranial pectoral

Musculocutaneous

Common peroneal

Axillary

Radial

Femoral

Ulnar

Caudal cutaneous
sural

Intercostals
(ventral branches spinal)

Lateral cutaneous antebrachial

Saphenous

Lateral thoracic

Superficial peroneal

Median

Caudal cutaneous
antebrachial

Deep peroneal

Medial cutaneous antebrachial

Ulnar

Lateral plantar

Dorsal branch
of ulnar

Medial dorsal metatarsal

Lateral palmar

Medial palmar

Lateral dorsal metatarsal

Medial plantar

Communicating branch

Medial plantar digital

Lateral plantar digital

Medial palmar digital

Dorsal branch of
lateral plantar digital

Lateral palmar digital

Dorsal branch of
lateral palmar digital

28

PLATE 1.27   Central and somatic nervous system of the stallion. Right lateral view.

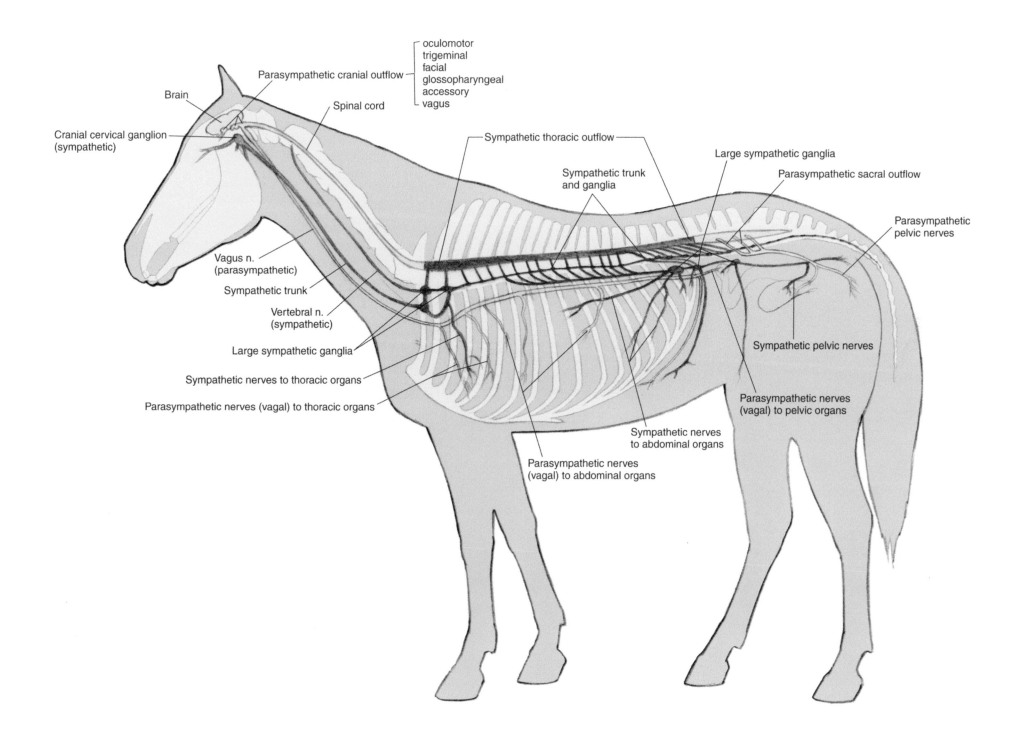

Brain

Parasympathetic cranial outflow ⎡ oculomotor
⎢ trigeminal
⎢ facial
⎢ glossopharyngeal
⎢ accessory
⎣ vagus

Spinal cord

Cranial cervical ganglion
(sympathetic)

Sympathetic thoracic outflow

Large sympathetic ganglia

Sympathetic trunk
and ganglia

Parasympathetic sacral outflow

Parasympathetic
pelvic nerves

Vagus n.
(parasympathetic)

Sympathetic trunk

Vertebral n.
(sympathetic)

Large sympathetic ganglia

Sympathetic pelvic nerves

Sympathetic nerves to thoracic organs

Parasympathetic nerves (vagal) to thoracic organs

Parasympathetic nerves
(vagal) to pelvic organs

Sympathetic nerves
to abdominal organs

Parasympathetic nerves
(vagal) to abdominal organs

29

PLATE 1.28   Autonomic nervous system of the mare.   Left lateral view. n = nerve

SECTION 2 THE OX *(Bos taurus,* also *Bos indicus)*

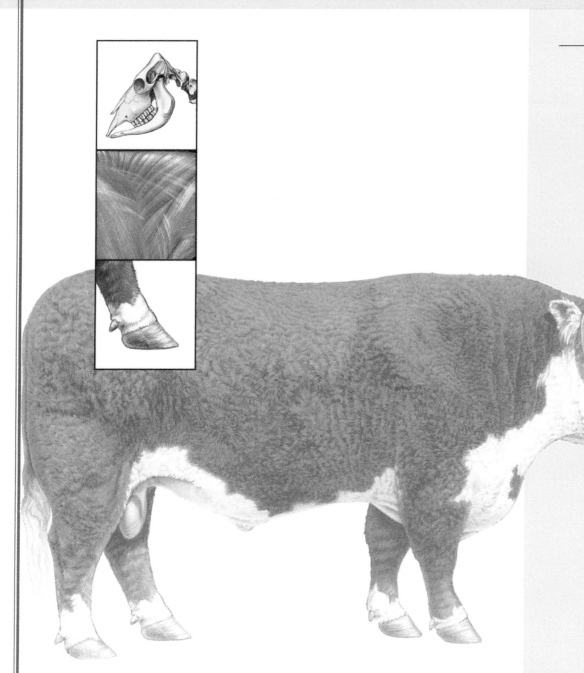

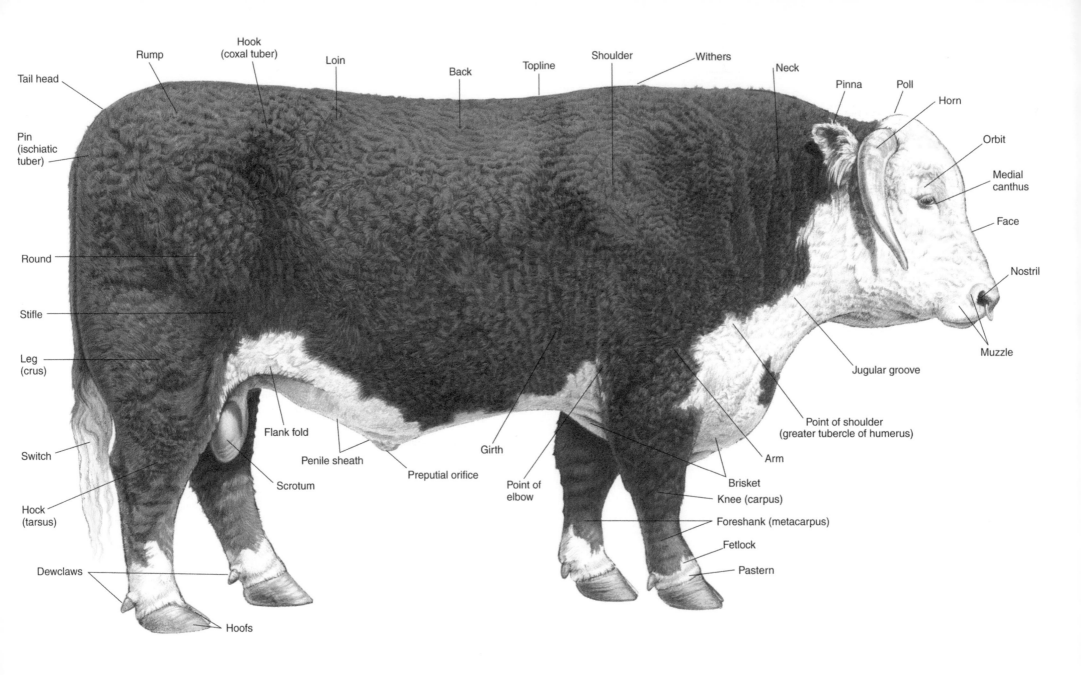

PLATE 2.1 Right lateral view of a beef bull.

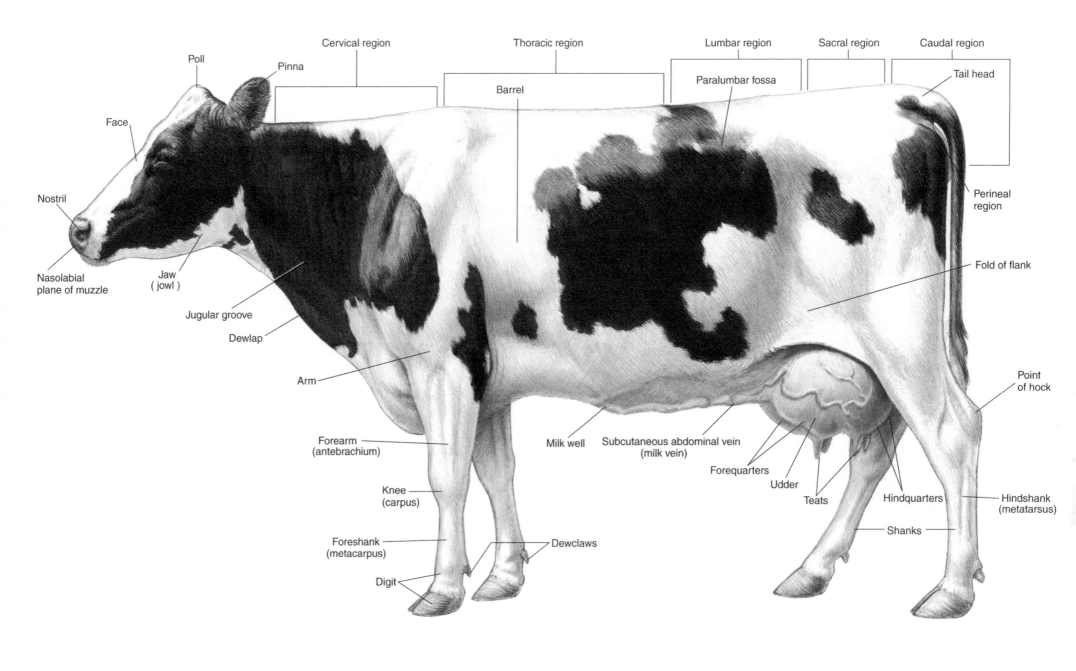

Cervical region

Thoracic region

Lumbar region

Sacral region

Caudal region

Poll

Pinna

Barrel

Paralumbar fossa

Tail head

Face

Nostril

Nasolabial
plane of muzzle

Jaw
(jowl)

Jugular groove

Dewlap

Arm

Perineal
region

Fold of flank

Point
of hock

Forearm
(antebrachium)

Milk well

Subcutaneous abdominal vein
(milk vein)

Forequarters

Udder

Hindquarters

Hindshank
(metatarsus)

Knee
(carpus)

Teats

Foreshank
(metacarpus)

Dewclaws

Shanks

Digit

33

PLATE 2.2   Left lateral view of a dairy cow. Dorsal vertebral regions indicated.

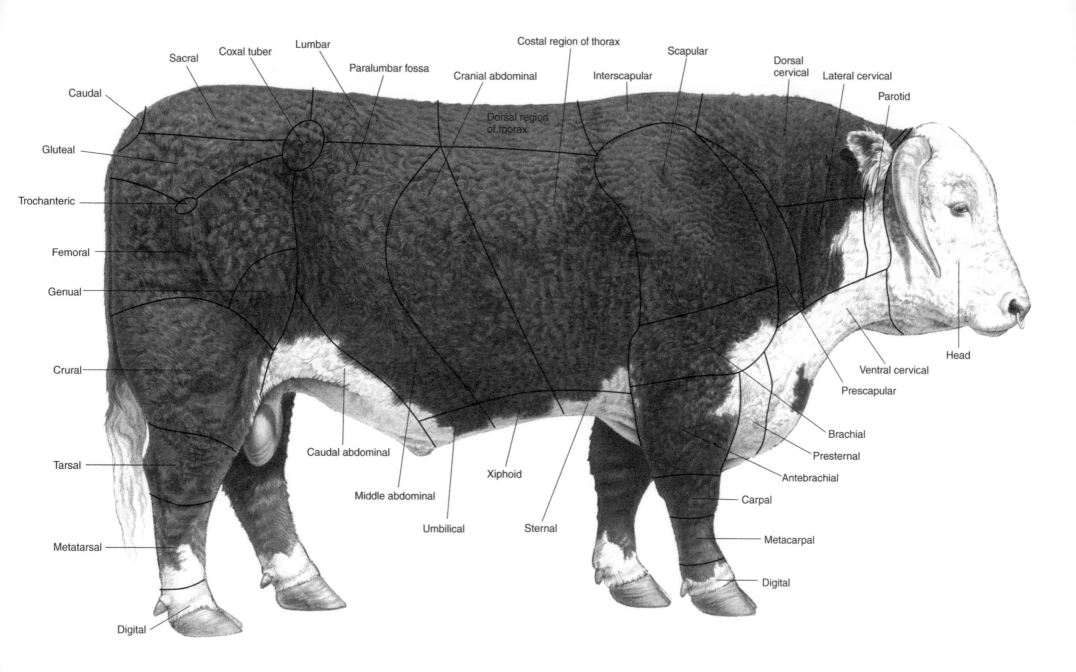

Caudal

Sacral

Coxal tuber

Lumbar

Paralumbar fossa

Costal region of thorax

Cranial abdominal

Dorsal region of thorax

Interscapular

Scapular

Dorsal cervical

Lateral cervical

Parotid

Gluteal

Trochanteric

Femoral

Genual

Crural

Tarsal

Metatarsal

Digital

Caudal abdominal

Middle abdominal

Umbilical

Xiphoid

Sternal

Head

Ventral cervical

Prescapular

Brachial

Presternal

Antebrachial

Carpal

Metacarpal

Digital

PLATE 2.3   Body regions of the ox. Right lateral view.

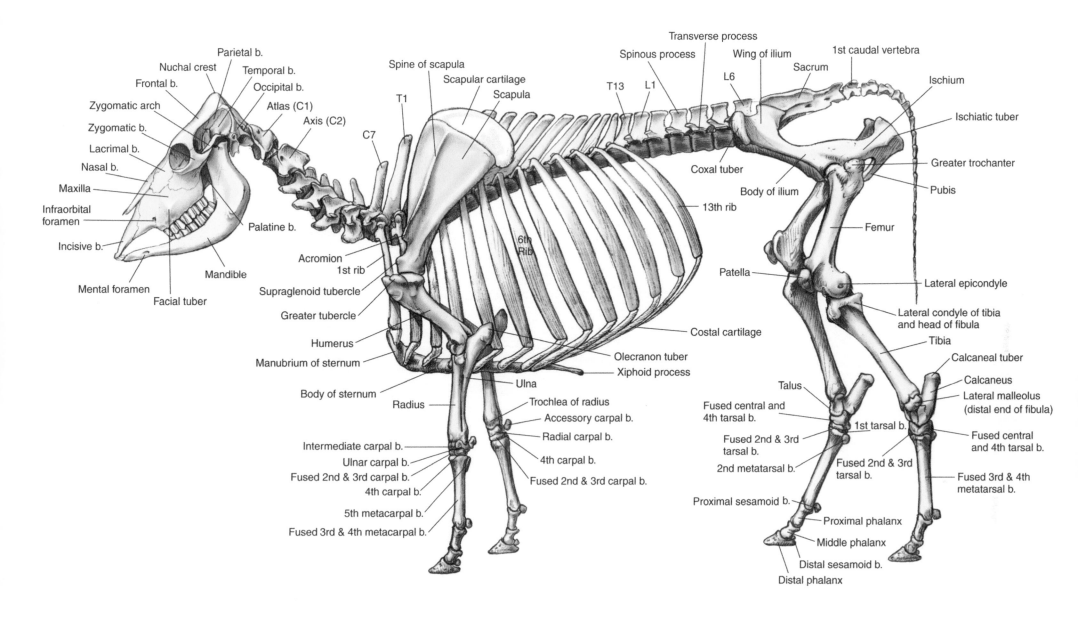

Parietal b.

Nuchal crest
Temporal b.

Frontal b.
Occipital b.

Zygomatic arch
Atlas (C1)

Zygomatic b.
Axis (C2)

Lacrimal b.

Nasal b.

Maxilla

Infraorbital
foramen

Incisive b.

Palatine b.

Mental foramen

Mandible

Facial tuber

Spine of scapula
Scapular cartilage
Scapula

Transverse process
Spinous process
Wing of ilium
Sacrum
1st caudal vertebra

T13
L1
L6
Ischium

Ischiatic tuber

Coxal tuber

Body of ilium

Greater trochanter

Pubis

13th rib

Femur

C7

T1

6th
Rib

Acromion

1st rib

Supraglenoid tubercle

Greater tubercle

Humerus

Manubrium of sternum

Body of sternum

Radius

Trochlea of radius

Accessory carpal b.

Radial carpal b.

4th carpal b.

Fused 2nd & 3rd carpal b.

Intermediate carpal b.

Ulnar carpal b.

Fused 2nd & 3rd carpal b.

4th carpal b.

5th metacarpal b.

Fused 3rd & 4th metacarpal b.

Costal cartilage

Olecranon tuber
Xiphoid process

Ulna

Patella

Lateral epicondyle

Lateral condyle of tibia
and head of fibula

Tibia

Calcaneal tuber

Calcaneus

Lateral malleolus
(distal end of fibula)

Talus

Fused central and
4th tarsal b.

Fused 2nd & 3rd
tarsal b.

2nd metatarsal b.

1st tarsal b.

Fused 2nd & 3rd
tarsal b.

Fused central
and 4th tarsal b.

Fused 3rd & 4th
metatarsal b.

Proximal sesamoid b.

Proximal phalanx

Middle phalanx

Distal sesamoid b.

Distal phalanx

35

PLATE 2.4   Skeleton of the ox. Left lateral view. C = cervical vertebra, T = thoracic vertebra,
L = lumbar vertebra, b = bone

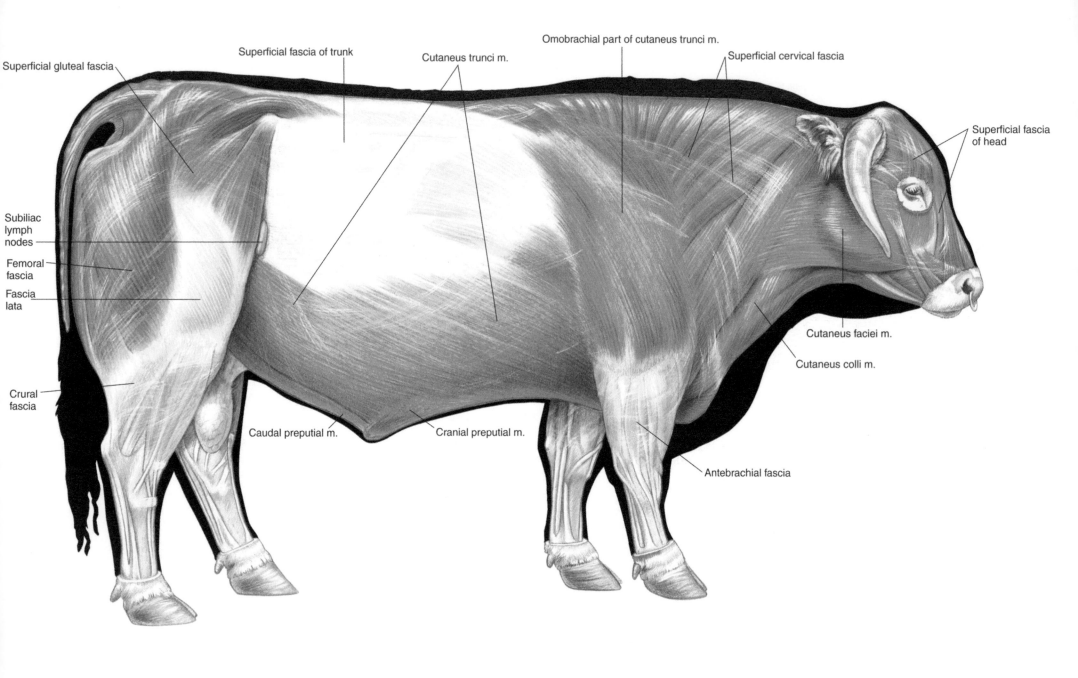

Superficial gluteal fascia

Superficial fascia of trunk

Cutaneus trunci m.

Omobrachial part of cutaneus trunci m.

Superficial cervical fascia

Superficial fascia of head

Subiliac lymph nodes

Femoral fascia

Fascia lata

Crural fascia

Caudal preputial m.

Cranial preputial m.

Antebrachial fascia

Cutaneus faciei m.

Cutaneus colli m.

36

PLATE 2.5 Cutaneous muscles and major fasciae of the bull. Right lateral view. n = nerve, m = muscle

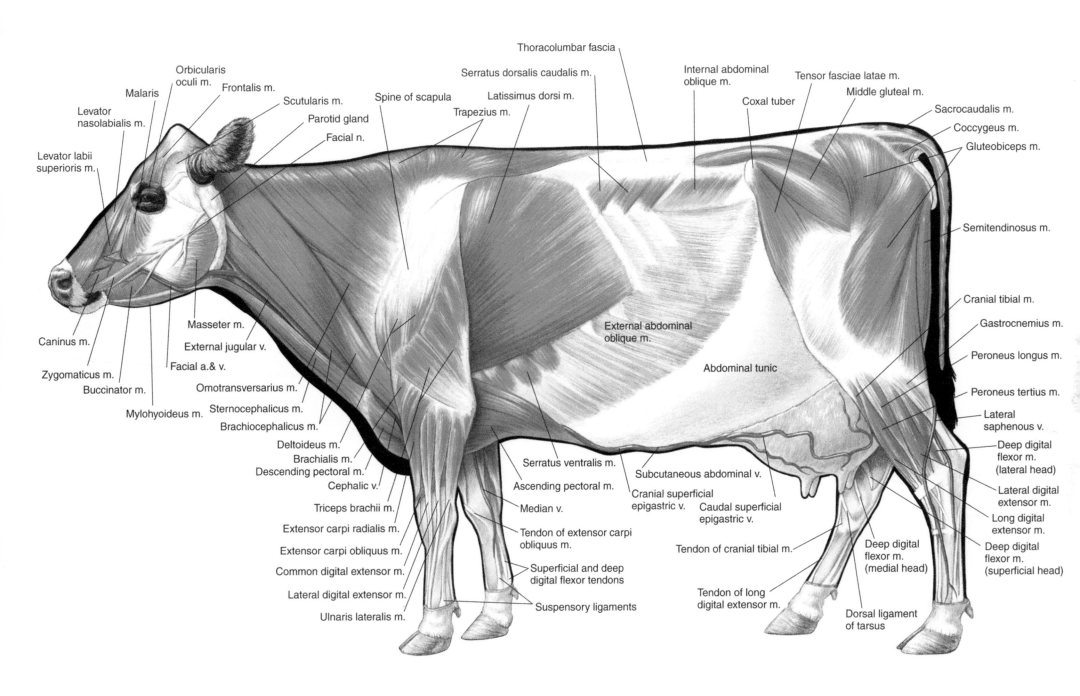

Levator
nasolabialis m.

Levator labii
superioris m.

Malaris

Orbicularis
oculi m.

Frontalis m.

Scutularis m.

Parotid gland

Facial n.

Spine of scapula

Trapezius m.

Thoracolumbar fascia

Serratus dorsalis caudalis m.

Latissimus dorsi m.

Internal abdominal
oblique m.

Coxal tuber

Tensor fasciae latae m.

Middle gluteal m.

Sacrocaudalis m.

Coccygeus m.

Gluteobiceps m.

Semitendinosus m.

Caninus m.

Zygomaticus m.

Buccinator m.

Mylohyoideus m.

Masseter m.

External jugular v.

Facial a.& v.

Omotransversarius m.

Sternocephalicus m.

Brachiocephalicus m.

Deltoideus m.

Brachialis m.

Descending pectoral m.

Cephalic v.

Triceps brachii m.

Extensor carpi radialis m.

Extensor carpi obliquus m.

Common digital extensor m.

Lateral digital extensor m.

Ulnaris lateralis m.

External abdominal
oblique m.

Abdominal tunic

Serratus ventralis m.

Ascending pectoral m.

Median v.

Tendon of extensor carpi
obliquus m.

Superficial and deep
digital flexor tendons

Suspensory ligaments

Subcutaneous abdominal v.

Cranial superficial
epigastric v.

Caudal superficial
epigastric v.

Tendon of cranial tibial m.

Tendon of long
digital extensor m.

Deep digital
flexor m.
(medial head)

Dorsal ligament
of tarsus

Cranial tibial m.

Gastrocnemius m.

Peroneus longus m.

Peroneus tertius m.

Lateral
saphenous v.

Deep digital
flexor m.
(lateral head)

Lateral digital
extensor m.

Long digital
extensor m.

Deep digital
flexor m.
(superficial head)

PLATE 2.6 Superficial muscles and veins of the cow. Left lateral view.
m = muscle, v = vein, a = artery, n = nerve

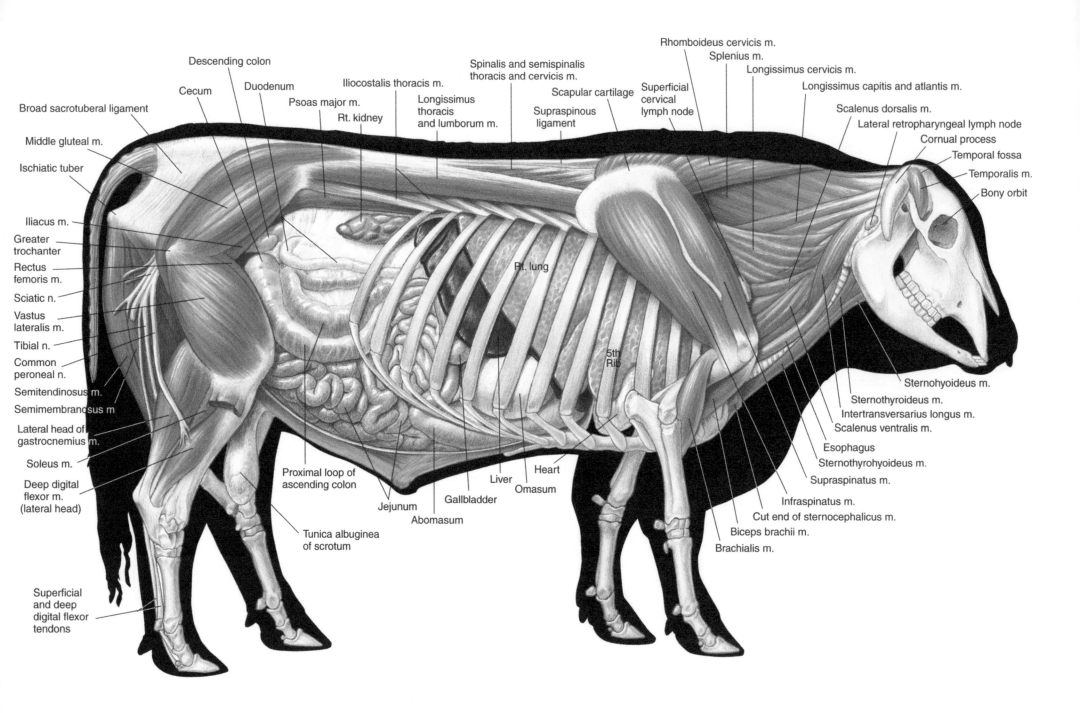

Rhomboideus cervicis m.

Spinalis and semispinalis
thoracis and cervicis m.

Splenius m.

Longissimus cervicis m.

Descending colon

Iliocostalis thoracis m.

Longissimus capitis and atlantis m.

Cecum

Duodenum

Scapular cartilage

Superficial
cervical
lymph node

Scalenus dorsalis m.

Broad sacrotuberal ligament

Psoas major m.

Longissimus
thoracis
and lumborum m.

Supraspinous
ligament

Lateral retropharyngeal lymph node

Rt. kidney

Suprascapular

Cornual process

Middle gluteal m.

Temporal fossa

Ischiatic tuber

Temporalis m.

Bony orbit

Iliacus m.

Greater
trochanter

Rectus
femoris m.

Rt. lung

Sciatic n.

Vastus
lateralis m.

Tibial n.

5th
Rib

Common
peroneal n.

Sternohyoideus m.

Semitendinosus m.

Sternothyroideus m.

Semimembranosus m

Intertransversarius longus m.

Scalenus ventralis m.

Lateral head of
gastrocnemius m.

Esophagus

Soleus m.

Sternothyrohyoideus m.

Proximal loop of
ascending colon

Heart

Supraspinatus m.

Deep digital
flexor m.
(lateral head)

Liver

Jejunum

Gallbladder

Omasum

Infraspinatus m.

Abomasum

Cut end of sternocephalicus m.

Tunica albuginea
of scrotum

Biceps brachii m.

Superficial
and deep
digital flexor
tendons

Brachialis m.

PLATE 2.7   Deep cervical muscles and *in situ* viscera of the bull. Greater
omentum removed. Right lateral view. m = muscle, n = nerve

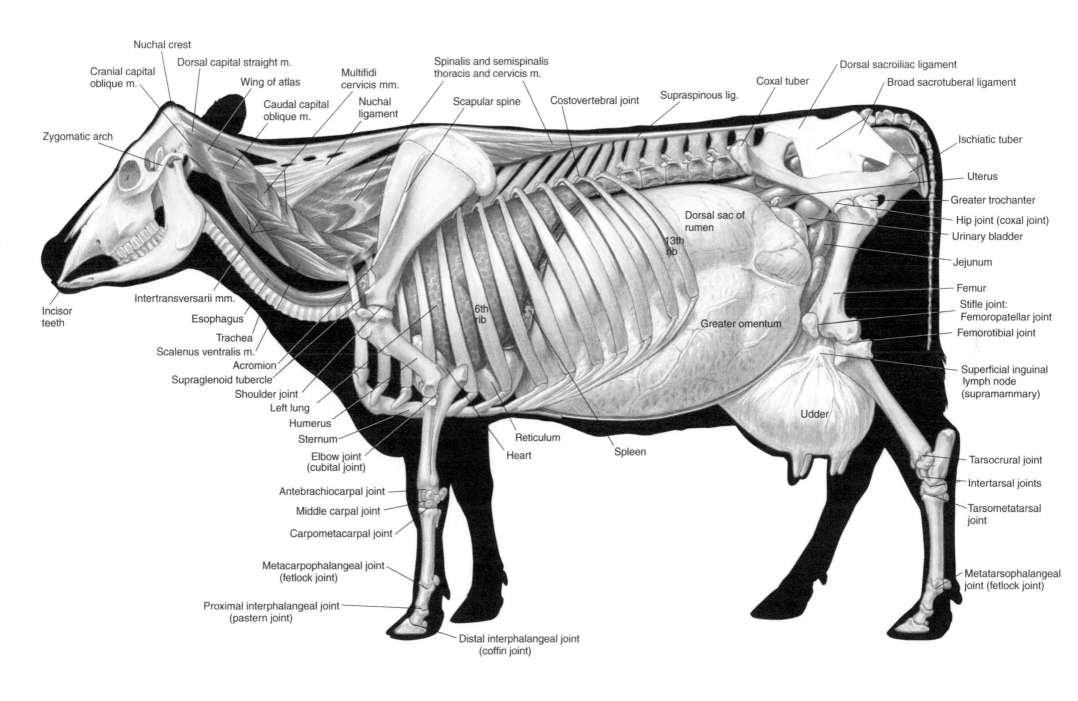

Nuchal crest

Cranial capital oblique m.

Dorsal capital straight m.

Wing of atlas

Caudal capital oblique m.

Multifidi cervicis mm.

Nuchal ligament

Spinalis and semispinalis thoracis and cervicis m.

Scapular spine

Costovertebral joint

Supraspinous lig.

Dorsal sacroiliac ligament

Coxal tuber

Broad sacrotuberal ligament

Zygomatic arch

Ischiatic tuber

Dorsal sac of rumen

Uterus

Greater trochanter

Hip joint (coxal joint)

Urinary bladder

13th rib

Jejunum

Femur

Stifle joint: Femoropatellar joint

Femorotibial joint

Incisor teeth

Intertransversarii mm.

Esophagus

Trachea

Scalenus ventralis m.

Acromion

Supraglenoid tubercle

Shoulder joint

Left lung

Humerus

Sternum

6th rib

Greater omentum

Superficial inguinal lymph node (supramammary)

Udder

Reticulum

Heart

Spleen

Elbow joint (cubital joint)

Tarsocrural joint

Intertarsal joints

Antebrachiocarpal joint

Middle carpal joint

Carpometacarpal joint

Tarsometatarsal joint

Metacarpophalangeal joint (fetlock joint)

Metatarsophalangeal joint (fetlock joint)

Proximal interphalangeal joint (pastern joint)

Distal interphalangeal joint (coffin joint)

39

PLATE 2.8 Deep cervical muscles, major joints, *in situ* viscera, and udder of the cow.
Left lateral view. m = muscle, lig = ligament

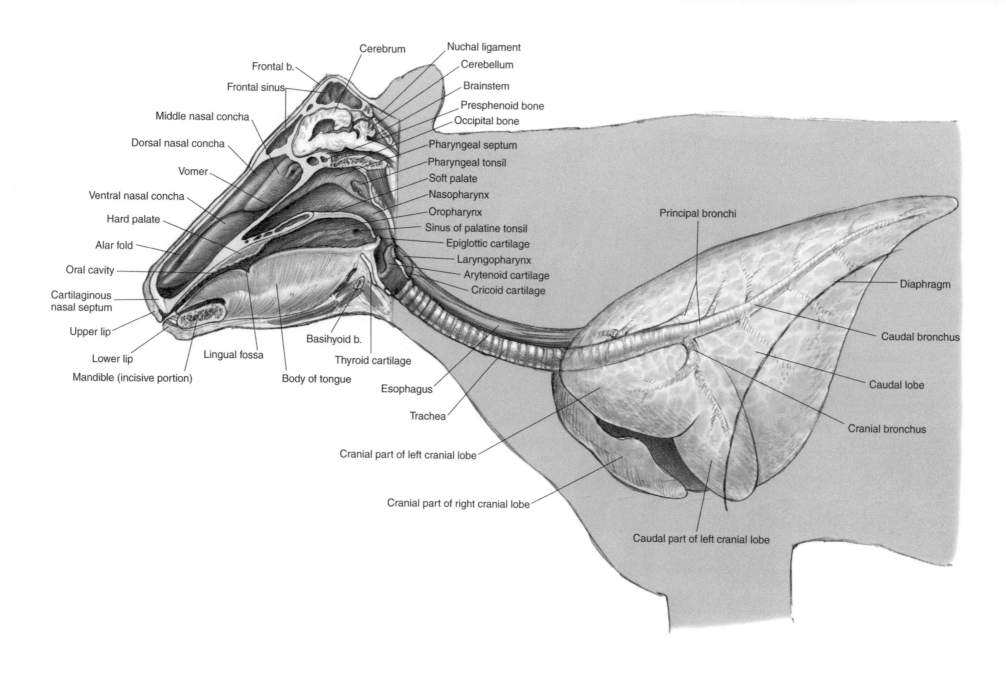

Cerebrum

Nuchal ligament

Frontal b.

Cerebellum

Frontal sinus

Brainstem

Middle nasal concha

Presphenoid bone

Dorsal nasal concha

Occipital bone

Vomer

Pharyngeal septum

Pharyngeal tonsil

Ventral nasal concha

Soft palate

Hard palate

Nasopharynx

Alar fold

Oropharynx

Oral cavity

Sinus of palatine tonsil

Epiglottic cartilage

Cartilaginous
nasal septum

Laryngopharynx

Arytenoid cartilage

Upper lip

Cricoid cartilage

Lower lip

Basihyoid b.

Mandible (incisive portion)

Thyroid cartilage

Lingual fossa

Body of tongue

Esophagus

Trachea

Principal bronchi

Diaphragm

Caudal bronchus

Caudal lobe

Cranial bronchus

Cranial part of left cranial lobe

Cranial part of right cranial lobe

Caudal part of left cranial lobe

40

PLATE 2.9   Median section of the head and left lateral view of the
respiratory system of the ox. b = bone

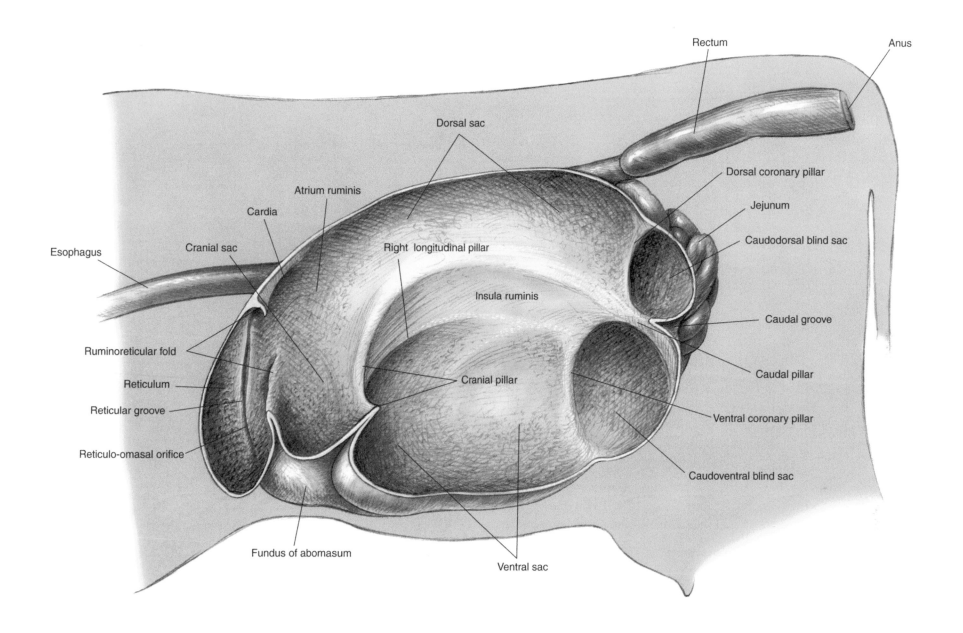

Rectum

Anus

Dorsal sac

Dorsal coronary pillar

Atrium ruminis

Jejunum

Cardia

Caudodorsal blind sac

Esophagus

Cranial sac

Right longitudinal pillar

Insula ruminis

Caudal groove

Ruminoreticular fold

Reticulum

Cranial pillar

Caudal pillar

Reticular groove

Ventral coronary pillar

Reticulo-omasal orifice

Caudoventral blind sac

Fundus of abomasum

Ventral sac

41

PLATE 2.10 Interior of the rumen and reticulum of the cow. Left lateral view.

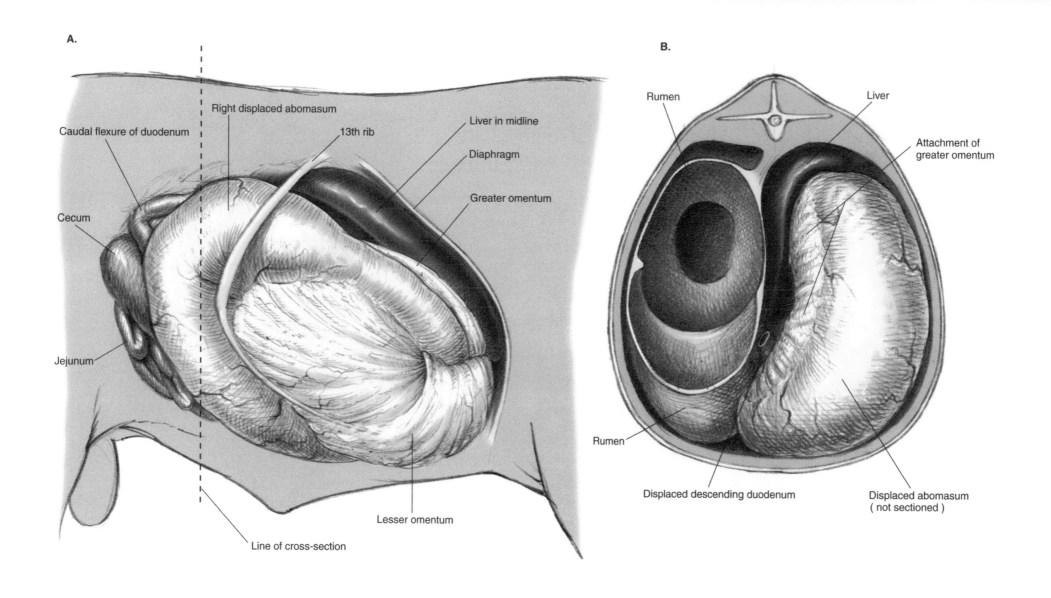

A.

Right displaced abomasum

Caudal flexure of duodenum

13th rib

Liver in midline

Cecum

Diaphragm

Greater omentum

Jejunum

Lesser omentum

Line of cross-section

B.

Rumen

Liver

Attachment of greater omentum

Rumen

Displaced descending duodenum

Displaced abomasum (not sectioned)

PLATE 2.11 Clinical condition: Right volvulus of the abomasum in a bull. **A.** Right lateral view. **B.** Cross-section. Caudocranial view. This problem occurs in cattle of varying types and ages. The long axis of the abomasum rotates dorsad and caudad, moving the greater curvature of the abomasum counterclockwise and toward the pelvis. This abnormal configuration displaces the liver mediad and draws the pyloric antrum and duodenum around the cranial aspect of the omasum.

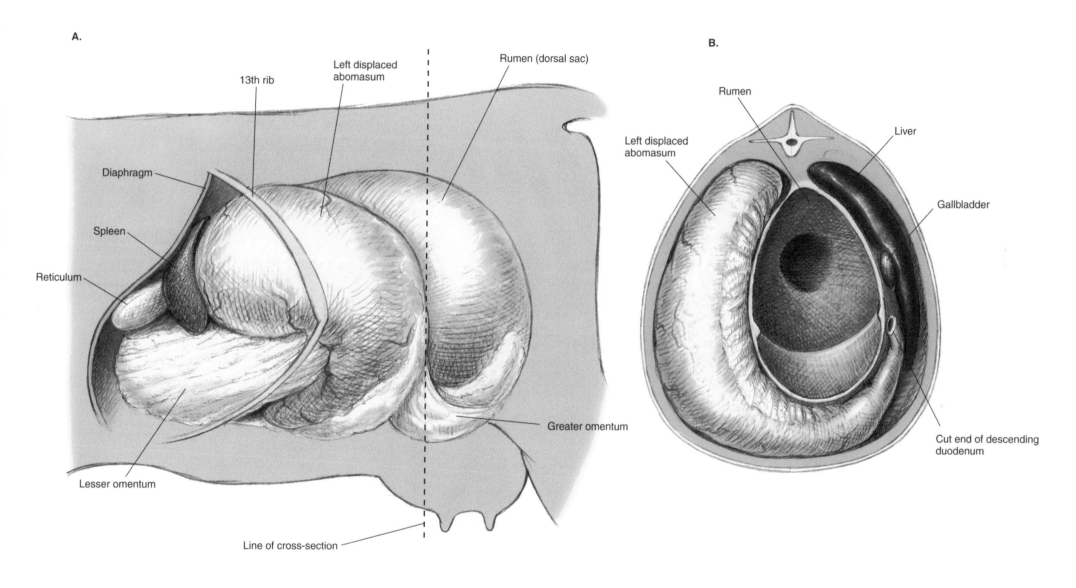

A.

13th rib

Left displaced abomasum

Rumen (dorsal sac)

B.

Rumen

Diaphragm

Spleen

Reticulum

Left displaced abomasum

Liver

Gallbladder

Lesser omentum

Greater omentum

Cut end of descending duodenum

Line of cross-section

PLATE 2.12   Clinical condition: Left displacement of the abomasum in a cow. **A.** Left lateral view.
B. Cross-section. Caudocranial view. This problem can occur commonly in lactating dairy
cattle during the first month postpartum and less frequently during other times
or in other types of cattle. The gas-filled abomasum moves to the left and
dorsad in the abdomen. It displaces the partially filled rumen
mediad and distorts the normal position and orientation of
the reticulum, omasum, and cranial rumen.

43

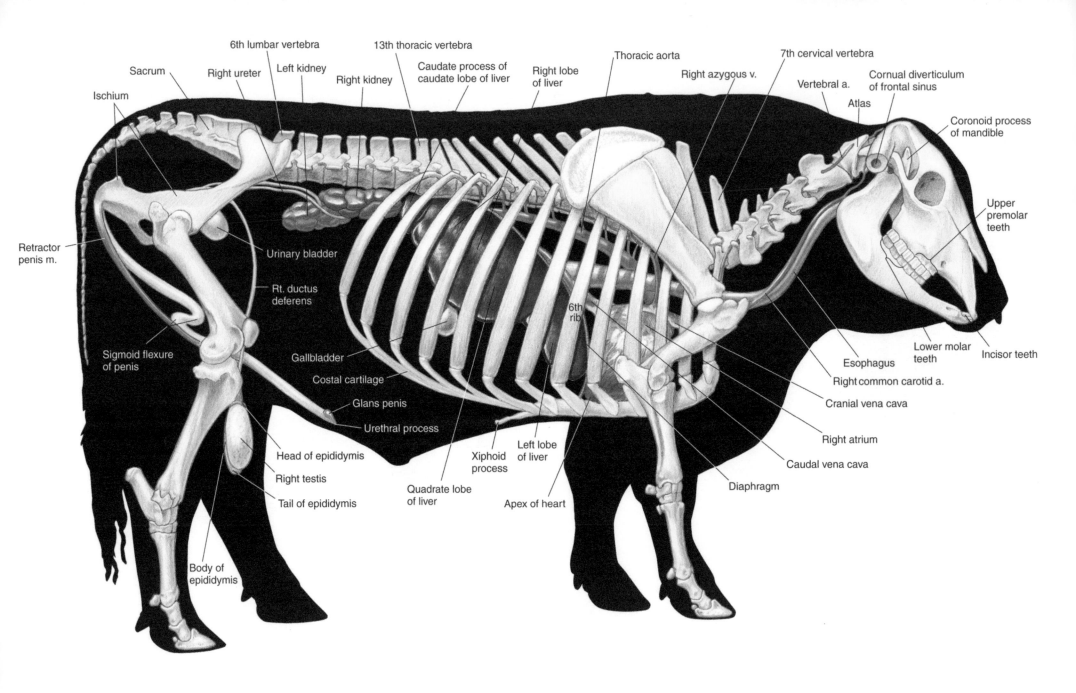

Ischium

Sacrum

Right ureter

6th lumbar vertebra

Left kidney

13th thoracic vertebra

Right kidney

Caudate process of caudate lobe of liver

Right lobe of liver

Thoracic aorta

Right azygous v.

7th cervical vertebra

Vertebral a.

Atlas

Cornual diverticulum of frontal sinus

Coronoid process of mandible

Upper premolar teeth

Retractor penis m.

Urinary bladder

Rt. ductus deferens

Sigmoid flexure of penis

Gallbladder

Costal cartilage

Glans penis

Urethral process

Head of epididymis

Right testis

Tail of epididymis

Body of epididymis

Xiphoid process

Quadrate lobe of liver

Apex of heart

Left lobe of liver

6th rib

Esophagus

Lower molar teeth

Incisor teeth

Right common carotid a.

Cranial vena cava

Right atrium

Caudal vena cava

Diaphragm

44

PLATE 2.13 Reproductive organs, urinary organs, liver, heart, and adjacent major vessels related to the skeleton of the bull. Stomach, intestines, and lungs are removed. Right lateral view. a = artery, v = vein, m = muscle

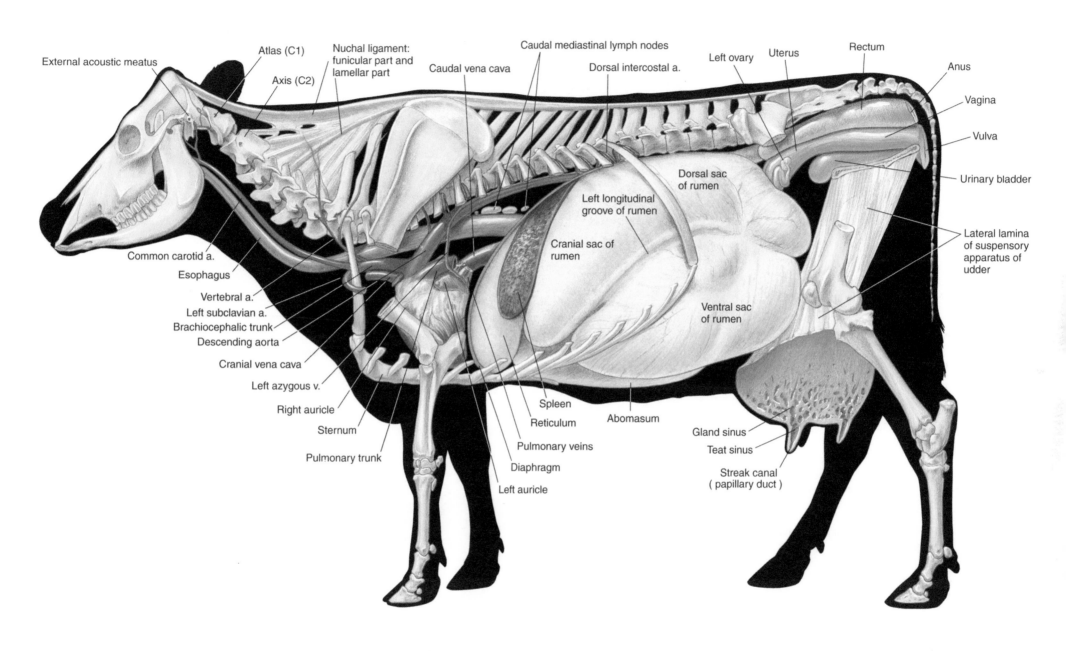

PLATE 2.14   Heart and adjacent major vessels, abdominal and pelvic viscera, and udder (mammary glands) of the cow. Lungs and intestines are removed. Left lateral view. v = vein, a = artery

45

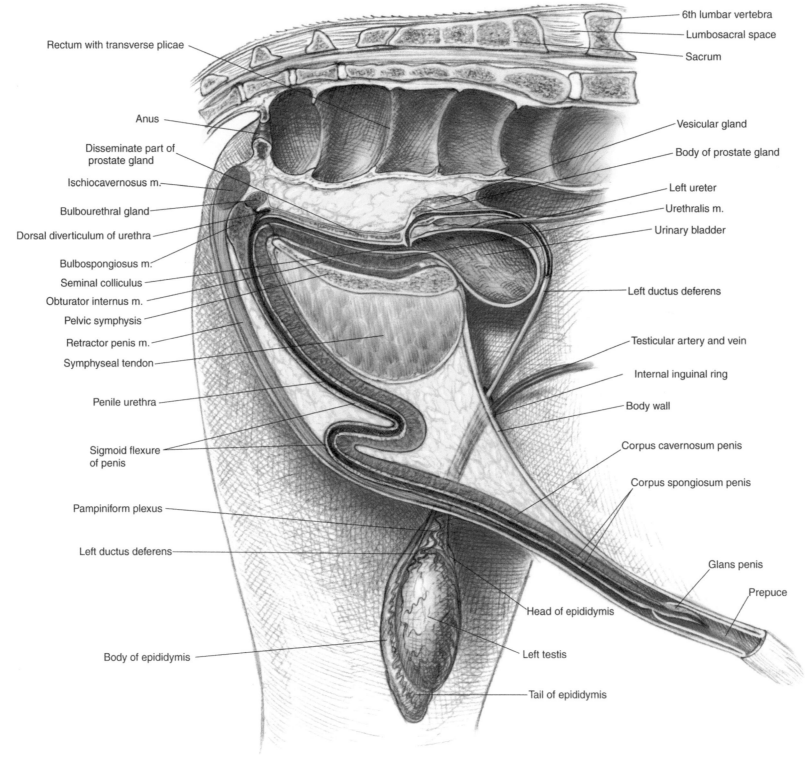

6th lumbar vertebra

Lumbosacral space

Sacrum

Rectum with transverse plicae

Anus

Disseminate part of prostate gland

Ischiocavernosus m.

Bulbourethral gland

Dorsal diverticulum of urethra

Bulbospongiosus m.

Seminal colliculus

Obturator internus m.

Pelvic symphysis

Retractor penis m.

Symphyseal tendon

Penile urethra

Sigmoid flexure of penis

Pampiniform plexus

Left ductus deferens

Body of epididymis

Vesicular gland

Body of prostate gland

Left ureter

Urethralis m.

Urinary bladder

Left ductus deferens

Testicular artery and vein

Internal inguinal ring

Body wall

Corpus cavernosum penis

Corpus spongiosum penis

Glans penis

Prepuce

Head of epididymis

Left testis

Tail of epididymis

46

PLATE 2.15 Relations of the reproductive organs of the bull. Median section. m = muscle

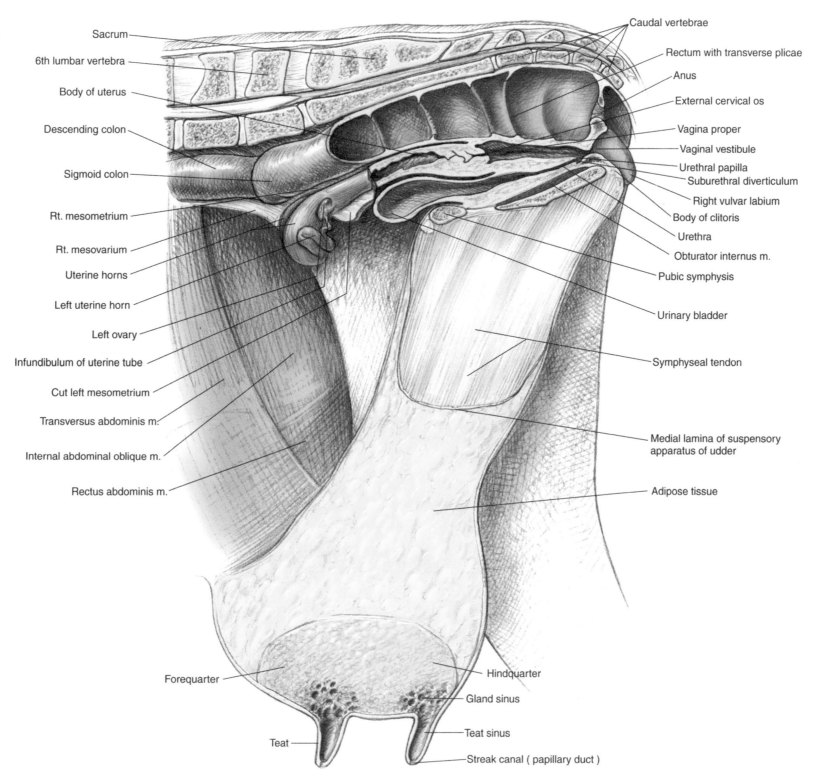

Sacrum

6th lumbar vertebra

Body of uterus

Descending colon

Sigmoid colon

Rt. mesometrium

Rt. mesovarium

Uterine horns

Left uterine horn

Left ovary

Infundibulum of uterine tube

Cut left mesometrium

Transversus abdominis m.

Internal abdominal oblique m.

Rectus abdominis m.

Forequarter

Teat

Caudal vertebrae

Rectum with transverse plicae

Anus

External cervical os

Vagina proper

Vaginal vestibule

Urethral papilla

Suburethral diverticulum

Right vulvar labium

Body of clitoris

Urethra

Obturator internus m.

Pubic symphysis

Urinary bladder

Symphyseal tendon

Medial lamina of suspensory apparatus of udder

Adipose tissue

Hindquarter

Gland sinus

Teat sinus

Streak canal (papillary duct)

47

PLATE 2.16   Relations of the reproductive organs of the cow. Median section. m = muscle

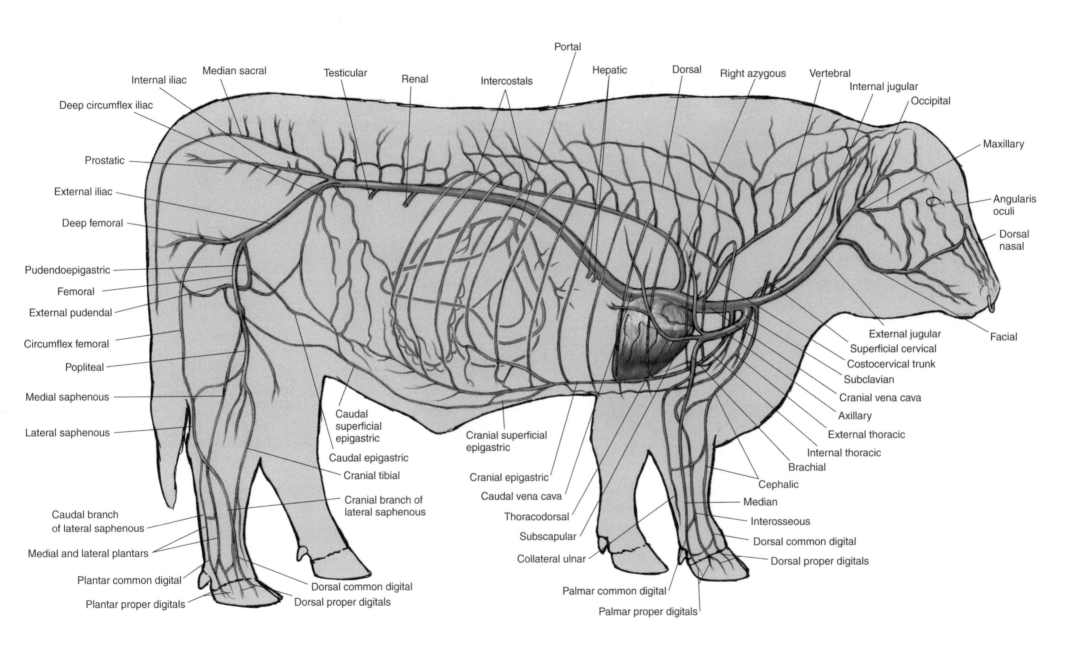

Internal iliac
Deep circumflex iliac
Median sacral
Testicular
Renal
Intercostals
Portal
Hepatic
Dorsal
Right azygous
Vertebral
Internal jugular
Occipital

Prostatic
Maxillary
External iliac
Deep femoral
Angularis oculi
Dorsal nasal

Pudendoepigastric
Femoral
External pudendal
Circumflex femoral
Popliteal
Medial saphenous
Lateral saphenous

External jugular
Superficial cervical
Costocervical trunk
Subclavian
Cranial vena cava
Axillary
External thoracic
Internal thoracic
Brachial
Cephalic
Median
Interosseous
Dorsal common digital
Dorsal proper digitals

Facial

Caudal superficial epigastric
Caudal epigastric
Cranial tibial
Cranial branch of lateral saphenous

Cranial superficial epigastric
Cranial epigastric
Caudal vena cava
Thoracodorsal
Subscapular
Collateral ulnar

Caudal branch of lateral saphenous
Medial and lateral plantars
Plantar common digital
Plantar proper digitals
Dorsal common digital
Dorsal proper digitals

Palmar common digital
Palmar proper digitals

PLATE 2.17 Major veins of the bull. Right lateral view.

48

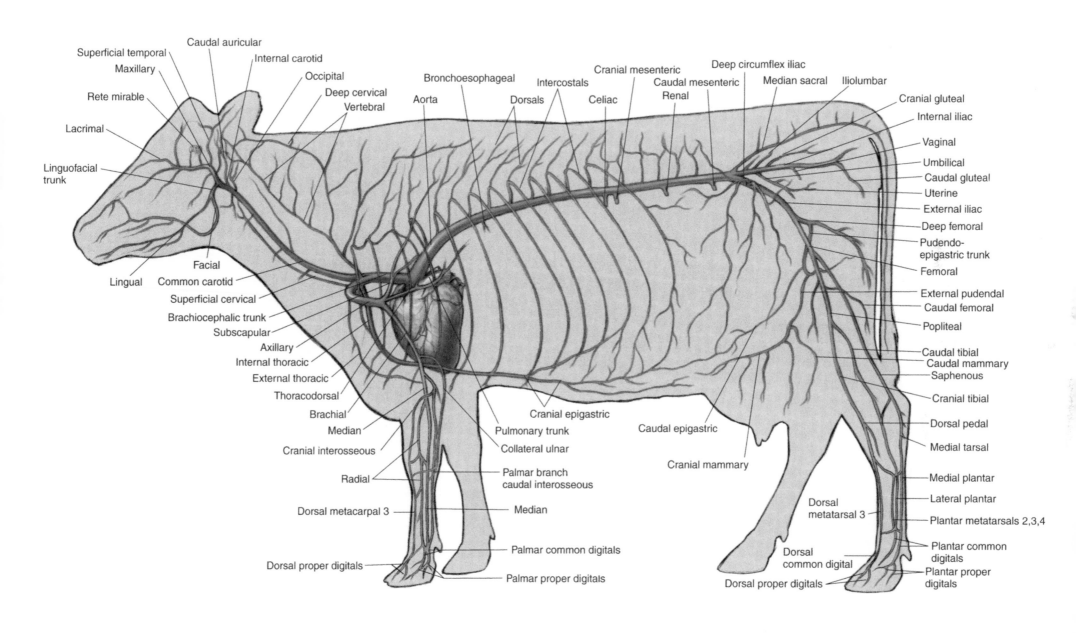

PLATE 2.18 Major arteries of the cow. Left lateral view.

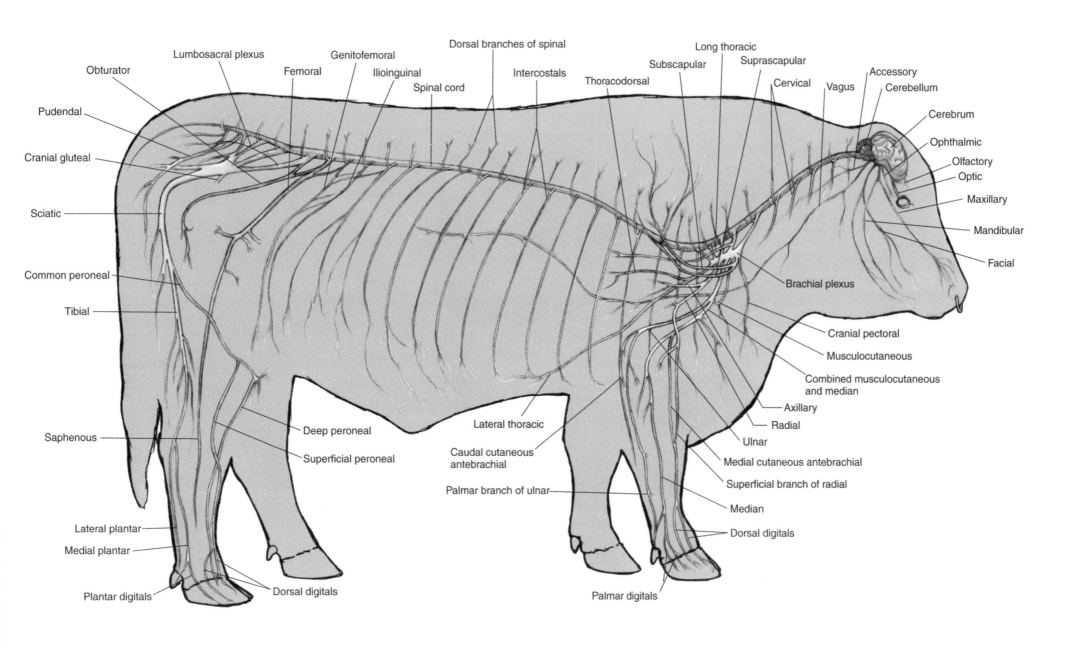

Obturator
Pudendal
Cranial gluteal
Sciatic
Common peroneal
Tibial
Saphenous
Lateral plantar
Medial plantar
Plantar digitals

Lumbosacral plexus
Femoral
Genitofemoral
Ilioinguinal
Spinal cord

Dorsal branches of spinal
Intercostals

Thoracodorsal

Long thoracic
Subscapular
Suprascapular
Cervical

Vagus

Accessory
Cerebellum
Cerebrum
Ophthalmic
Olfactory
Optic
Maxillary
Mandibular
Facial

Brachial plexus

Cranial pectoral
Musculocutaneous
Combined musculocutaneous
and median
Axillary
Radial
Ulnar
Medial cutaneous antebrachial
Superficial branch of radial
Median

Deep peroneal
Superficial peroneal

Lateral thoracic

Caudal cutaneous
antebrachial

Palmar branch of ulnar

Dorsal digitals

Palmar digitals

Dorsal digitals

PLATE 2.19   Central nervous system and principal nerves of the
peripheral nervous system of the bull. Right lateral view.

50

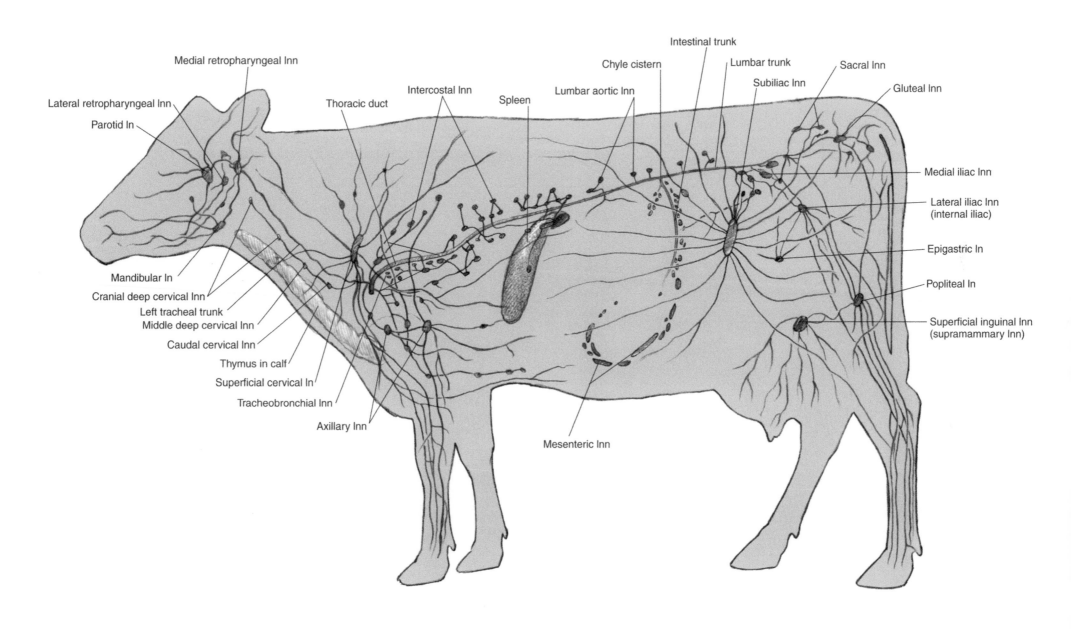

PLATE 2.20 Significant lymphatic organs of the cow. Left lateral view. ln = lymph node

Medial retropharyngeal lnn

Lateral retropharyngeal lnn

Parotid ln

Mandibular ln

Cranial deep cervical lnn

Left tracheal trunk

Middle deep cervical lnn

Caudal cervical lnn

Thymus in calf

Superficial cervical ln

Tracheobronchial lnn

Axillary lnn

Intercostal lnn

Thoracic duct

Spleen

Lumbar aortic lnn

Chyle cistern

Intestinal trunk

Lumbar trunk

Subiliac lnn

Sacral lnn

Gluteal lnn

Medial iliac lnn

Lateral iliac lnn
(internal iliac)

Epigastric ln

Popliteal ln

Superficial inguinal lnn
(supramammary lnn)

Mesenteric lnn

51

SECTION 3 THE SHEEP (*Ovis aries*)

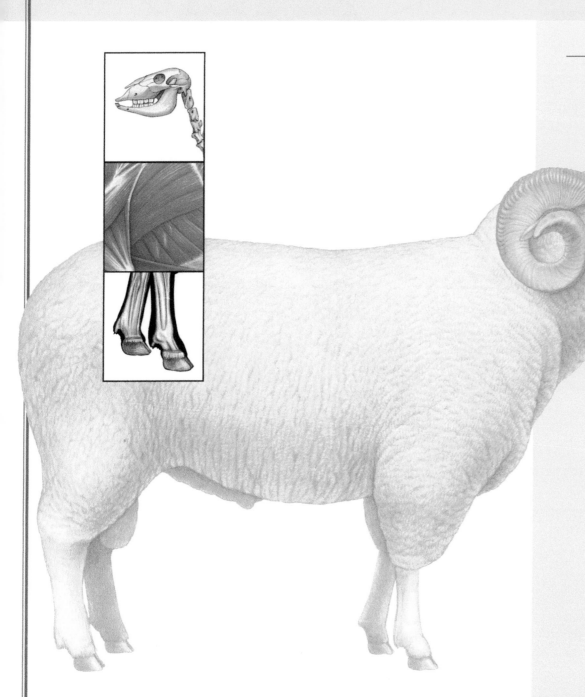

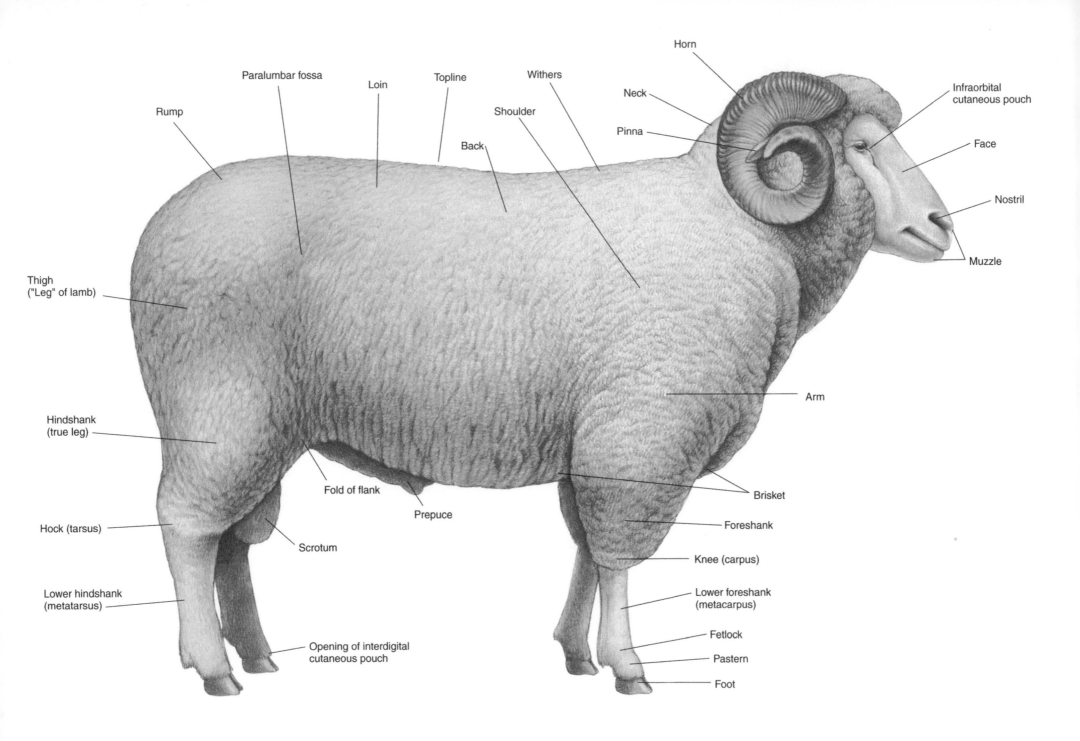

Horn

Infraorbital
cutaneous pouch

Neck

Paralumbar fossa

Loin

Topline

Withers

Pinna

Face

Rump

Shoulder

Nostril

Back

Muzzle

Thigh
("Leg" of lamb)

Arm

Hindshank
(true leg)

Brisket

Fold of flank

Foreshank

Hock (tarsus)

Prepuce

Knee (carpus)

Scrotum

Lower hindshank
(metatarsus)

Lower foreshank
(metacarpus)

Fetlock

Opening of interdigital
cutaneous pouch

Pastern

Foot

54

PLATE 3.1 Right lateral view of a ram.

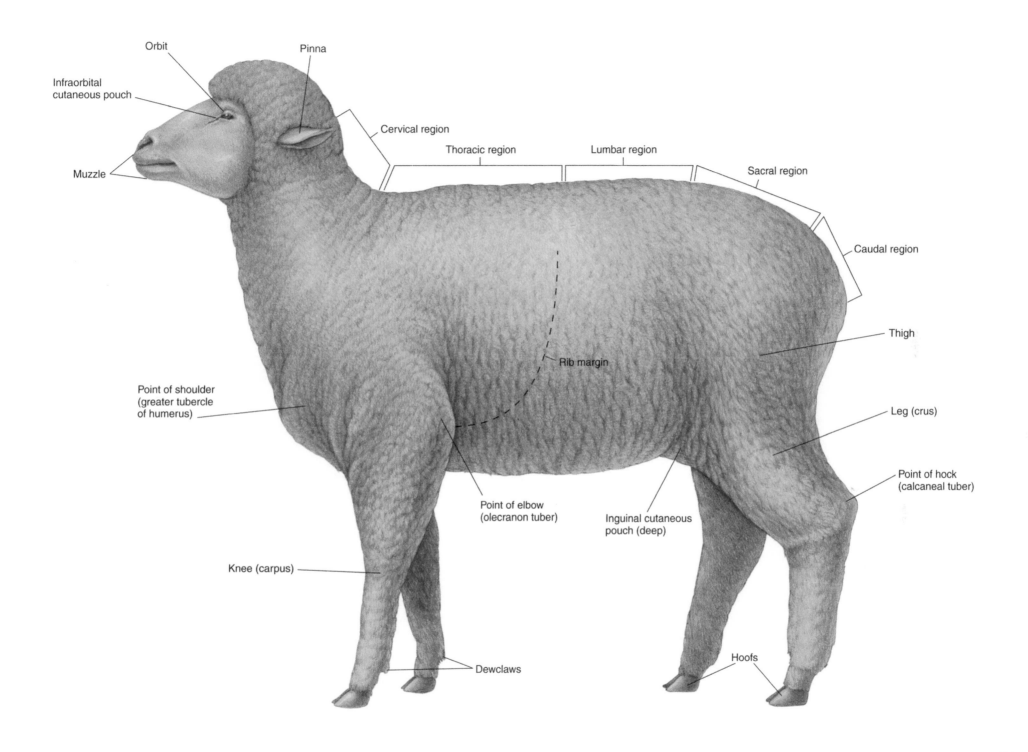

Orbit

Pinna

Infraorbital
cutaneous pouch

Cervical region

Thoracic region

Lumbar region

Sacral region

Muzzle

Caudal region

Rib margin

Thigh

Point of shoulder
(greater tubercle
of humerus)

Leg (crus)

Point of hock
(calcaneal tuber)

Point of elbow
(olecranon tuber)

Inguinal cutaneous
pouch (deep)

Knee (carpus)

Dewclaws

Hoofs

PLATE 3.2 Left lateral view of an ewe.

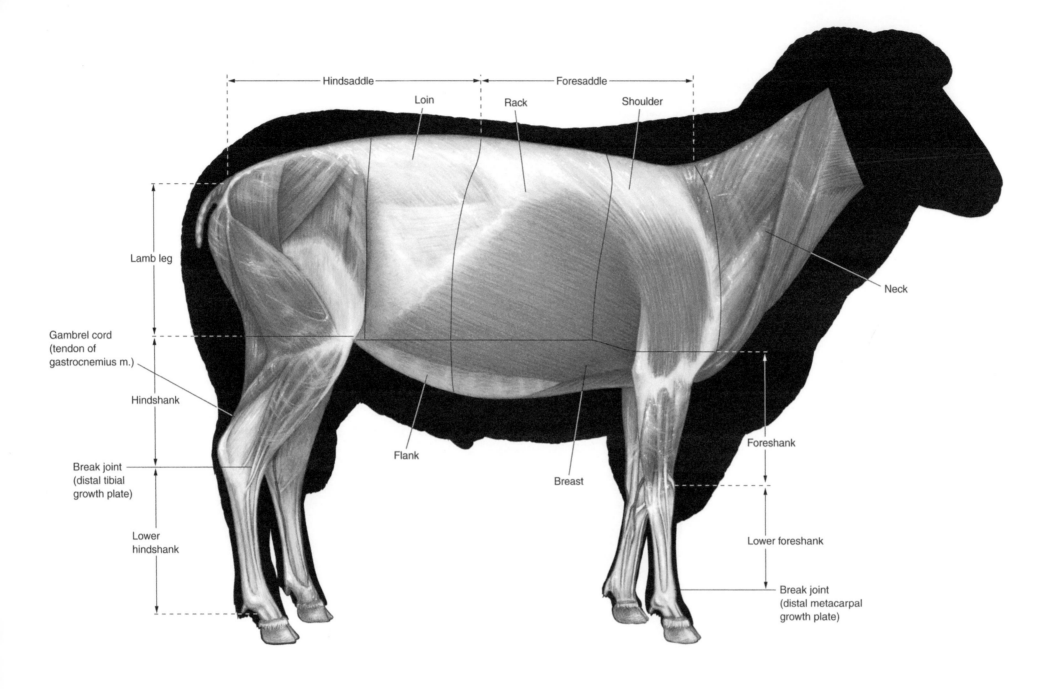

Hindsaddle

Foresaddle

Loin

Rack

Shoulder

Lamb leg

Neck

Gambrel cord
(tendon of
gastrocnemius m.)

Hindshank

Break joint
(distal tibial
growth plate)

Flank

Foreshank

Breast

Lower
hindshank

Lower foreshank

Break joint
(distal metacarpal
growth plate)

PLATE 3.3   Carcass cuts of the lamb. m = muscle

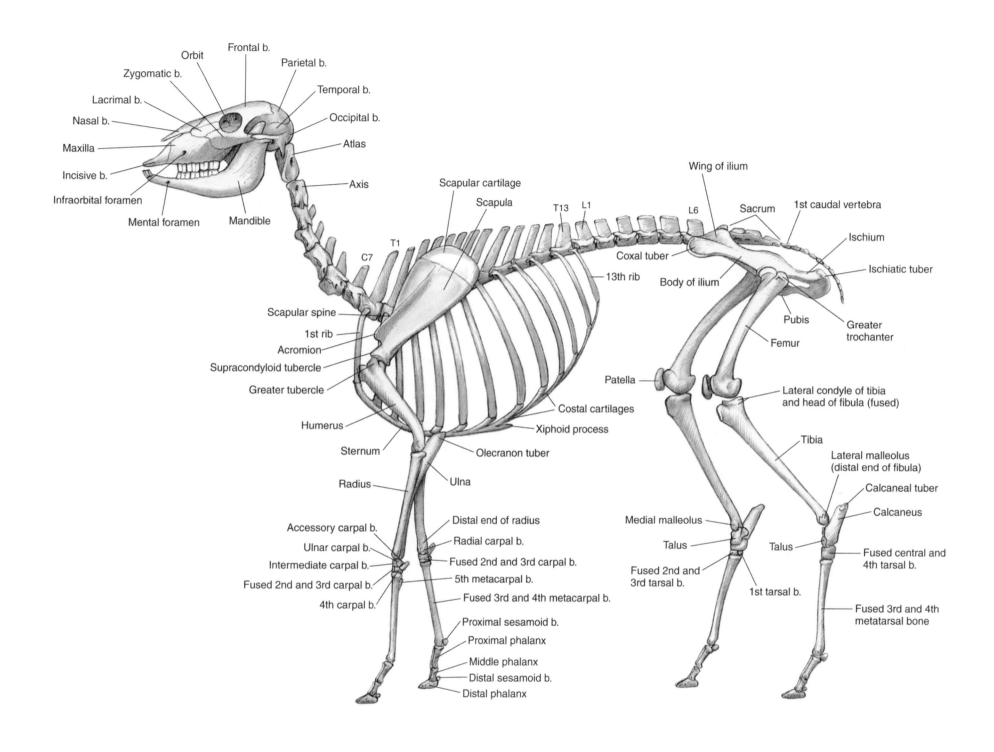

Orbit
Frontal b.
Parietal b.
Zygomatic b.
Temporal b.
Lacrimal b.
Occipital b.
Nasal b.
Atlas
Maxilla
Axis
Incisive b.
Infraorbital foramen
Mental foramen
Mandible

Scapular cartilage
Scapula
T13 L1
L6
Wing of ilium
Sacrum
1st caudal vertebra
Coxal tuber
Ischium
T1
13th rib
Body of ilium
Ischiatic tuber
C7
Scapular spine
Pubis
Greater trochanter
1st rib
Acromion
Femur
Supracondyloid tubercle
Greater tubercle
Patella
Lateral condyle of tibia and head of fibula (fused)
Humerus
Costal cartilages
Tibia
Sternum
Xiphoid process
Lateral malleolus (distal end of fibula)
Olecranon tuber
Radius
Ulna
Calcaneal tuber
Distal end of radius
Medial malleolus
Calcaneus
Accessory carpal b.
Radial carpal b.
Ulnar carpal b.
Talus
Talus
Fused central and 4th tarsal b.
Fused 2nd and 3rd carpal b.
Intermediate carpal b.
Fused 2nd and 3rd tarsal b.
Fused 2nd and 3rd carpal b.
5th metacarpal b.
1st tarsal b.
4th carpal b.
Fused 3rd and 4th metacarpal b.
Proximal sesamoid b.
Fused 3rd and 4th metatarsal bone
Proximal phalanx
Middle phalanx
Distal sesamoid b.
Distal phalanx

PLATE 3.4   Skeleton of the sheep. b = bone, C = cervical vertebra,
T = thoracic vertebra, L = lumbar vertebra

57

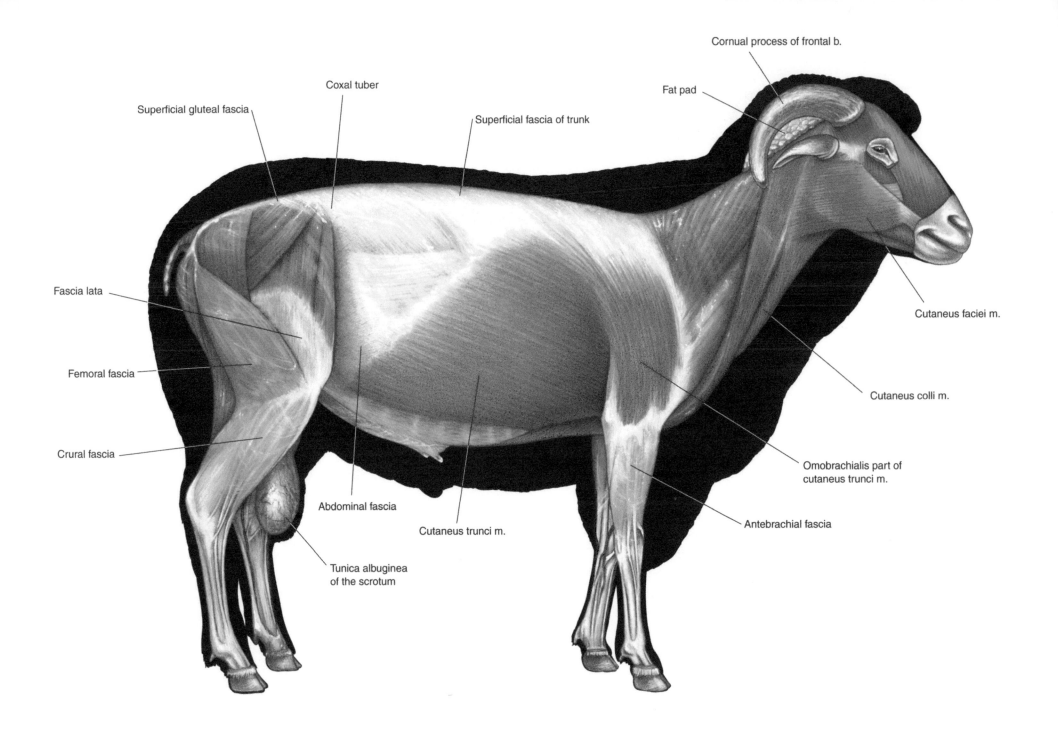

Cornual process of frontal b.

Fat pad

Coxal tuber

Superficial fascia of trunk

Superficial gluteal fascia

Cutaneus faciei m.

Fascia lata

Cutaneus colli m.

Femoral fascia

Omobrachialis part of
cutaneus trunci m.

Crural fascia

Abdominal fascia

Antebrachial fascia

Cutaneus trunci m.

Tunica albuginea
of the scrotum

58

PLATE 3.5   Cutaneous muscles and major fasciae of the ram.
Right lateral view. m = muscle, b = bone

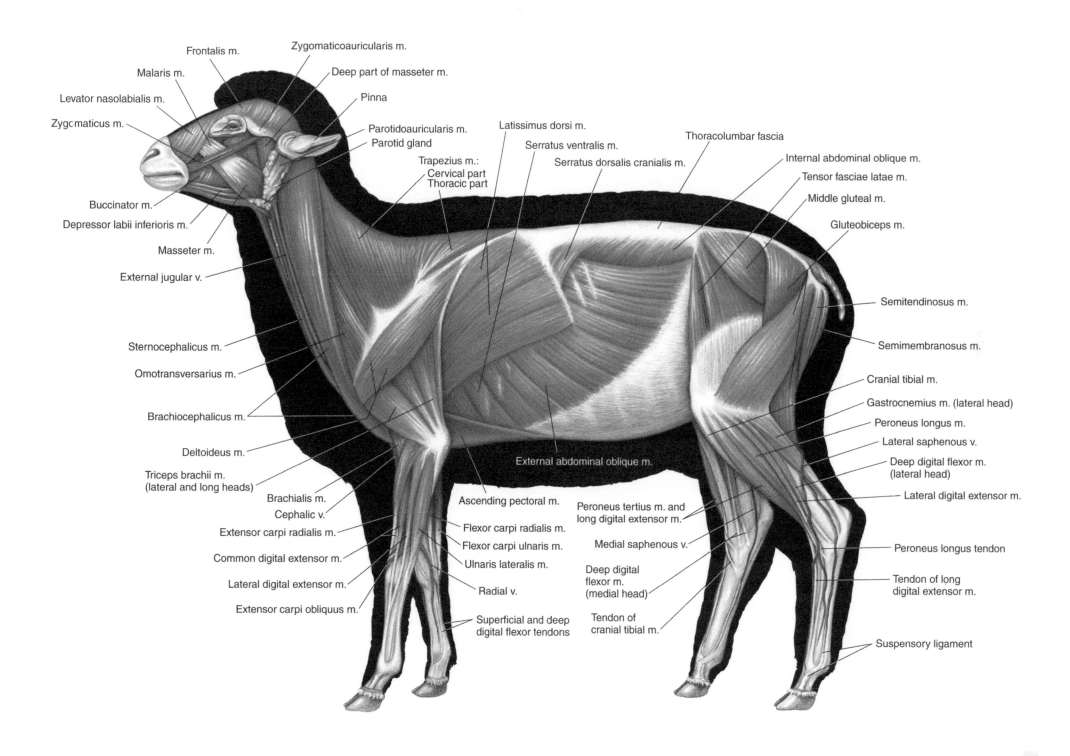

Frontalis m.

Zygomaticoauricularis m.

Malaris m.

Deep part of masseter m.

Levator nasolabialis m.

Pinna

Zygomaticus m.

Parotidoauricularis m.

Parotid gland

Latissimus dorsi m.

Serratus ventralis m.

Thoracolumbar fascia

Trapezius m.:
Cervical part
Thoracic part

Serratus dorsalis cranialis m.

Internal abdominal oblique m.

Tensor fasciae latae m.

Middle gluteal m.

Gluteobiceps m.

Buccinator m.

Depressor labii inferioris m.

Masseter m.

External jugular v.

Semitendinosus m.

Sternocephalicus m.

Semimembranosus m.

Omotransversarius m.

Cranial tibial m.

Brachiocephalicus m.

Gastrocnemius m. (lateral head)

Peroneus longus m.

Deltoideus m.

Lateral saphenous v.

External abdominal oblique m.

Deep digital flexor m.
(lateral head)

Triceps brachii m.
(lateral and long heads)

Lateral digital extensor m.

Brachialis m.

Cephalic v.

Ascending pectoral m.

Peroneus tertius m. and
long digital extensor m.

Peroneus longus tendon

Extensor carpi radialis m.

Flexor carpi radialis m.

Medial saphenous v.

Common digital extensor m.

Flexor carpi ulnaris m.

Tendon of long
digital extensor m.

Lateral digital extensor m.

Ulnaris lateralis m.

Deep digital
flexor m.
(medial head)

Extensor carpi obliquus m.

Radial v.

Superficial and deep
digital flexor tendons

Tendon of
cranial tibial m.

Suspensory ligament

59

PLATE 3.6 Superficial muscles and veins of the ewe. Left lateral view. m = muscle, v = vein

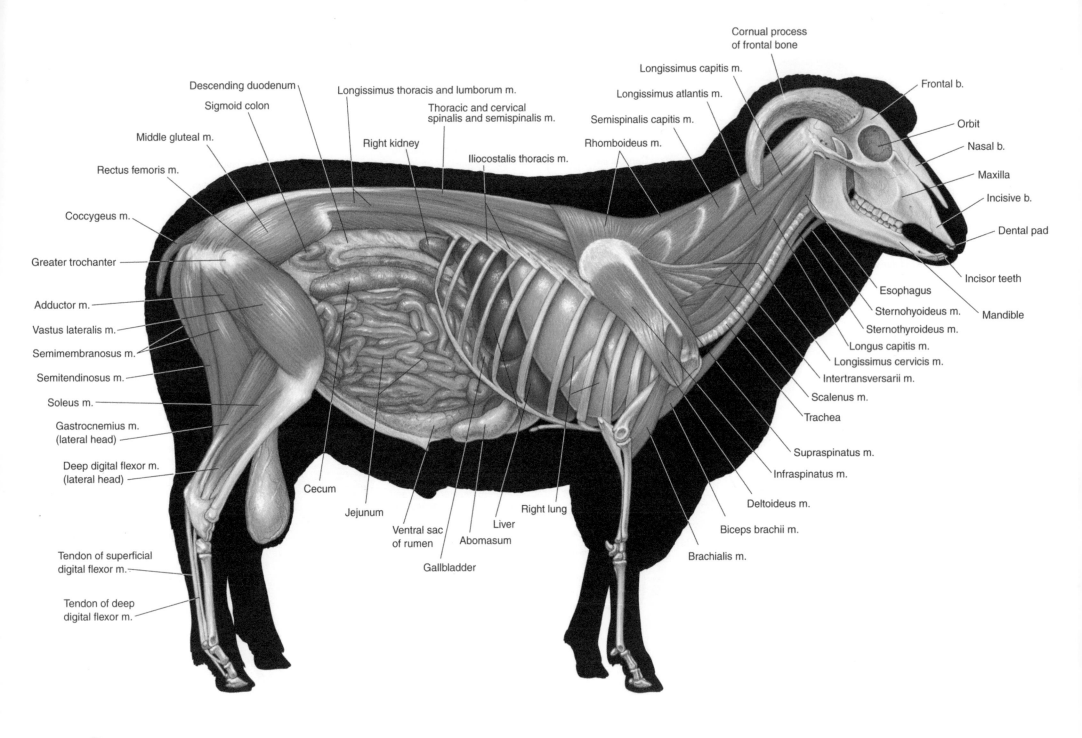

Cornual process
of frontal bone

Longissimus capitis m.

Descending duodenum

Longissimus thoracis and lumborum m.

Longissimus atlantis m.

Frontal b.

Sigmoid colon

Thoracic and cervical
spinalis and semispinalis m.

Semispinalis capitis m.

Orbit

Middle gluteal m.

Right kidney

Rhomboideus m.

Nasal b.

Rectus femoris m.

Iliocostalis thoracis m.

Maxilla

Incisive b.

Coccygeus m.

Dental pad

Greater trochanter

Incisor teeth

Esophagus

Adductor m.

Sternohyoideus m.

Vastus lateralis m.

Mandible

Semimembranosus m.

Sternothyroideus m.

Longus capitis m.

Semitendinosus m.

Longissimus cervicis m.

Soleus m.

Intertransversarii m.

Scalenus m.

Gastrocnemius m.
(lateral head)

Trachea

Deep digital flexor m.
(lateral head)

Supraspinatus m.

Cecum

Infraspinatus m.

Jejunum

Right lung

Deltoideus m.

Ventral sac
of rumen

Liver

Tendon of superficial
digital flexor m.

Abomasum

Biceps brachii m.

Gallbladder

Brachialis m.

Tendon of deep
digital flexor m.

60

PLATE 3.7 Deep cervical muscles and *in situ* viscera of the ram. Omentum removed.
Right lateral view. m = muscle, b = bone

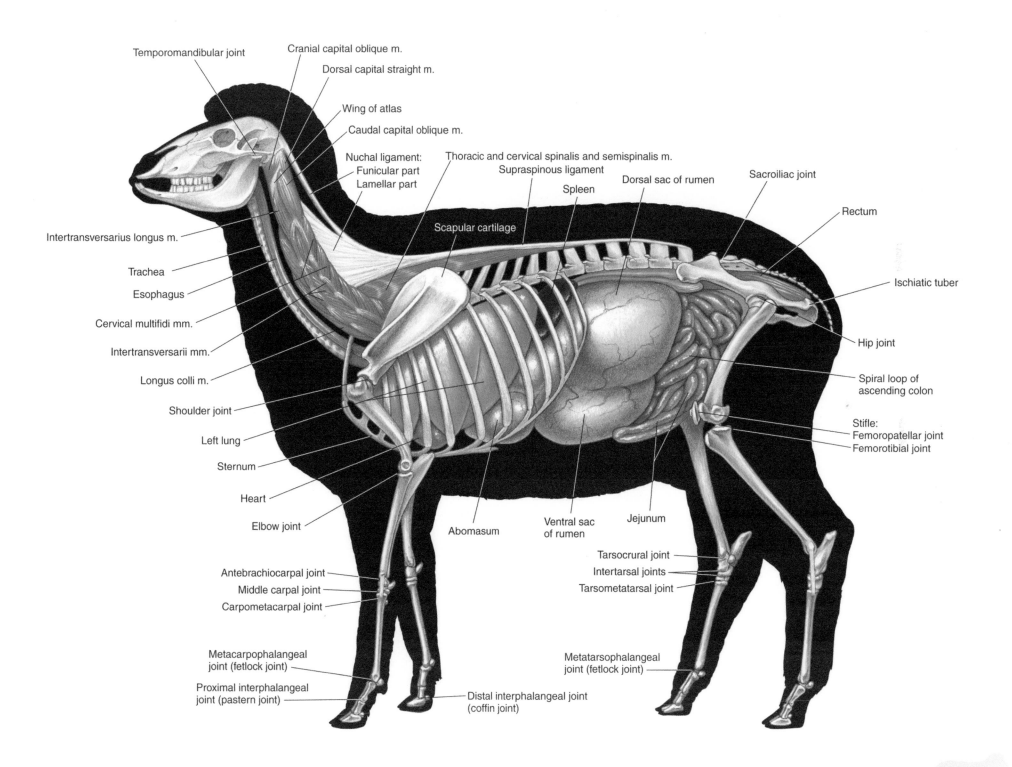

Temporomandibular joint

Cranial capital oblique m.

Dorsal capital straight m.

Wing of atlas

Caudal capital oblique m.

Nuchal ligament:
Funicular part
Lamellar part

Thoracic and cervical spinalis and semispinalis m.

Supraspinous ligament

Spleen

Dorsal sac of rumen

Sacroiliac joint

Rectum

Scapular cartilage

Intertransversarius longus m.

Trachea

Esophagus

Cervical multifidi mm.

Intertransversarii mm.

Longus colli m.

Shoulder joint

Left lung

Sternum

Heart

Elbow joint

Ischiatic tuber

Hip joint

Spiral loop of
ascending colon

Stifle:
Femoropatellar joint
Femorotibial joint

Abomasum

Ventral sac
of rumen

Jejunum

Tarsocrural joint

Intertarsal joints

Tarsometatarsal joint

Antebrachiocarpal joint

Middle carpal joint

Carpometacarpal joint

Metacarpophalangeal
joint (fetlock joint)

Proximal interphalangeal
joint (pastern joint)

Distal interphalangeal joint
(coffin joint)

Metatarsophalangeal
joint (fetlock joint)

PLATE 3.8   Deep cervical muscles, *in situ* viscera, skeleton, and major
joints of the ewe. Left lateral view. m = muscle

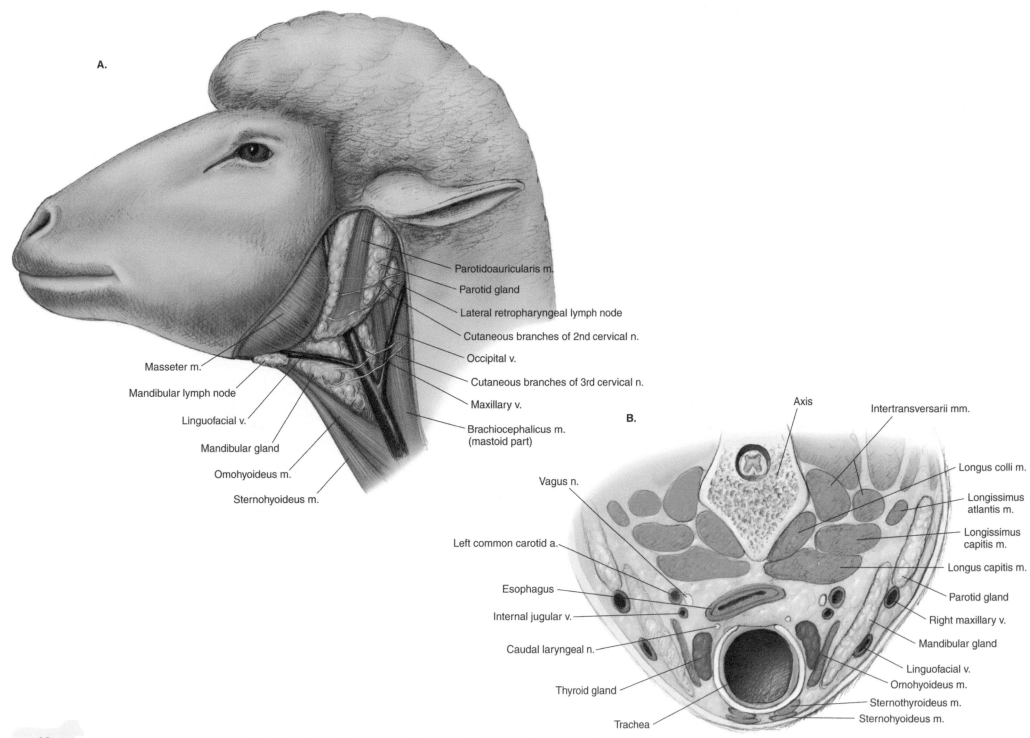

A.

Parotidoauricularis m.

Parotid gland

Lateral retropharyngeal lymph node

Cutaneous branches of 2nd cervical n.

Occipital v.

Cutaneous branches of 3rd cervical n.

Maxillary v.

Brachiocephalicus m.
(mastoid part)

Masseter m.

Mandibular lymph node

Linguofacial v.

Mandibular gland

Omohyoideus m.

Sternohyoideus m.

B.

Axis

Intertransversarii mm.

Longus colli m.

Longissimus atlantis m.

Longissimus capitis m.

Longus capitis m.

Parotid gland

Right maxillary v.

Mandibular gland

Linguofacial v.

Omohyoideus m.

Sternothyroideus m.

Sternohyoideus m.

Vagus n.

Left common carotid a.

Esophagus

Internal jugular v.

Caudal laryngeal n.

Thyroid gland

Trachea

62

PLATE 3.9   **A.** Dissection of the parotid region of a sheep. Skin, cutaneous muscles, and fascia are removed. Left lateral view. **B.** Cross-section of the neck at the level of the thyroid gland. Caudocranial view. m = muscle, v = vein, a = artery, n = nerve

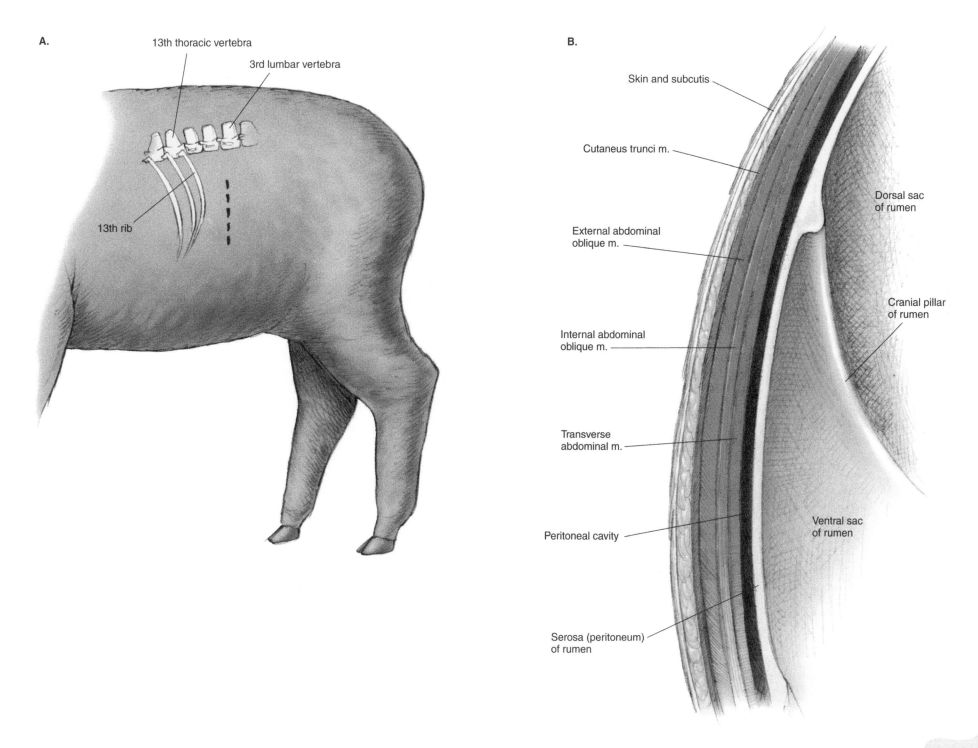

A.

13th thoracic vertebra

3rd lumbar vertebra

13th rib

B.

Skin and subcutis

Cutaneus trunci m.

External abdominal oblique m.

Internal abdominal oblique m.

Transverse abdominal m.

Peritoneal cavity

Serosa (peritoneum) of rumen

Dorsal sac of rumen

Cranial pillar of rumen

Ventral sac of rumen

PLATE 3.10   A. Location of the left flank incision: *dashed line*. **B.** Cross-section through the left abdominal wall and subjacent ruminal wall. Caudocranial view. m = muscle

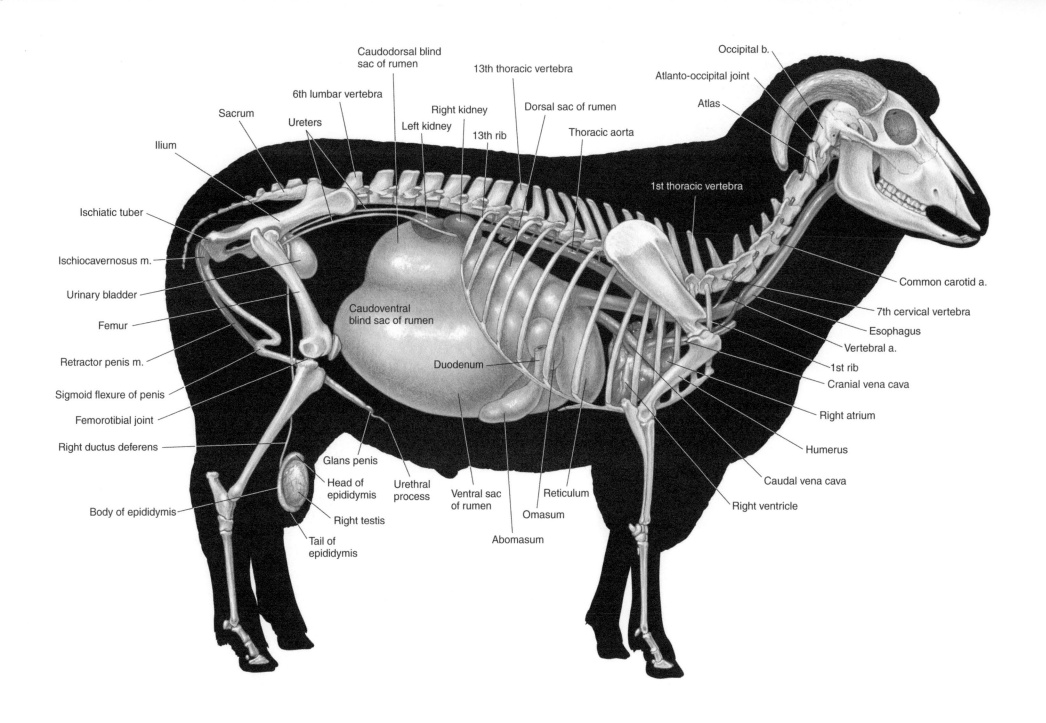

Occipital b.

Atlanto-occipital joint

Caudodorsal blind
sac of rumen

13th thoracic vertebra

Atlas

6th lumbar vertebra

Right kidney

Dorsal sac of rumen

Sacrum

Ureters

Left kidney

13th rib

Thoracic aorta

Ilium

1st thoracic vertebra

Ischiatic tuber

Common carotid a.

Ischiocavernosus m.

7th cervical vertebra

Urinary bladder

Esophagus

Caudoventral
blind sac of rumen

Vertebral a.

Femur

Duodenum

1st rib

Retractor penis m.

Cranial vena cava

Sigmoid flexure of penis

Right atrium

Femorotibial joint

Right ductus deferens

Humerus

Glans penis

Caudal vena cava

Head of
epididymis

Urethral
process

Ventral sac
of rumen

Reticulum

Right ventricle

Body of epididymis

Right testis

Omasum

Tail of
epididymis

Abomasum

PLATE 3.11 Reproductive organs, urinary organs, esophagus and stomach, heart, and
adjacent major vessels related to the skeleton of the ram. Right lateral view.
b = bone, m = muscle, a = artery

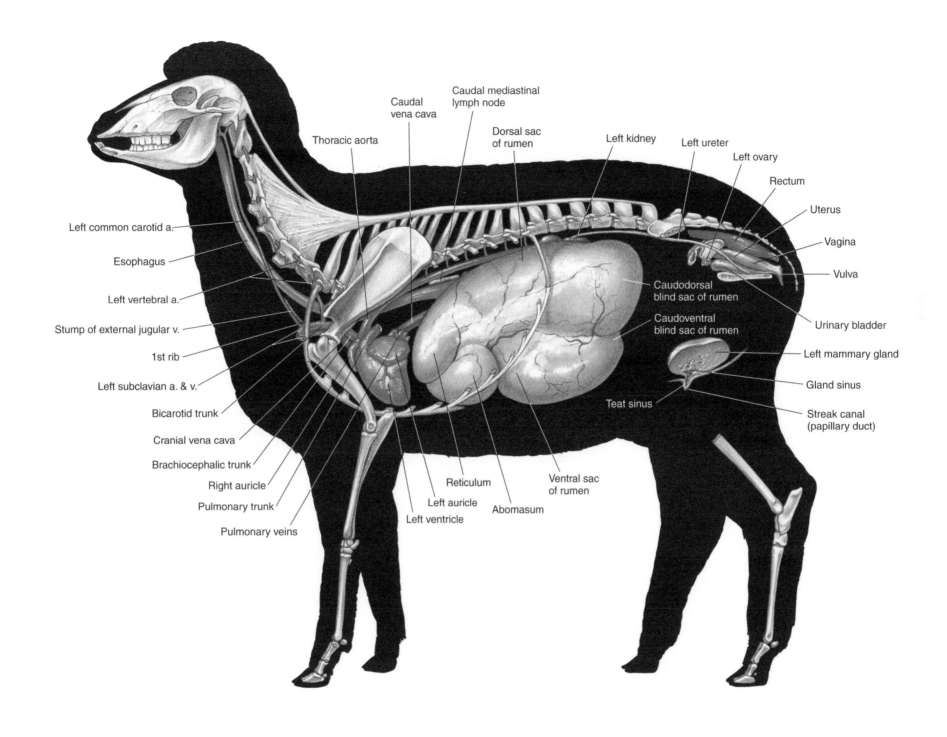

Caudal vena cava

Caudal mediastinal lymph node

Thoracic aorta

Dorsal sac of rumen

Left kidney

Left ureter

Left ovary

Rectum

Uterus

Vagina

Vulva

Left common carotid a.

Esophagus

Left vertebral a.

Stump of external jugular v.

1st rib

Left subclavian a. & v.

Bicarotid trunk

Cranial vena cava

Brachiocephalic trunk

Right auricle

Pulmonary trunk

Pulmonary veins

Caudodorsal blind sac of rumen

Caudoventral blind sac of rumen

Urinary bladder

Left mammary gland

Gland sinus

Teat sinus

Streak canal (papillary duct)

Reticulum

Left auricle

Left ventricle

Ventral sac of rumen

Abomasum

PLATE 3.12   Reproductive organs, urinary organs, heart, and adjacent major vessels, esophagus and stomach of the ewe. Left lateral view. a = artery, v =vein

65

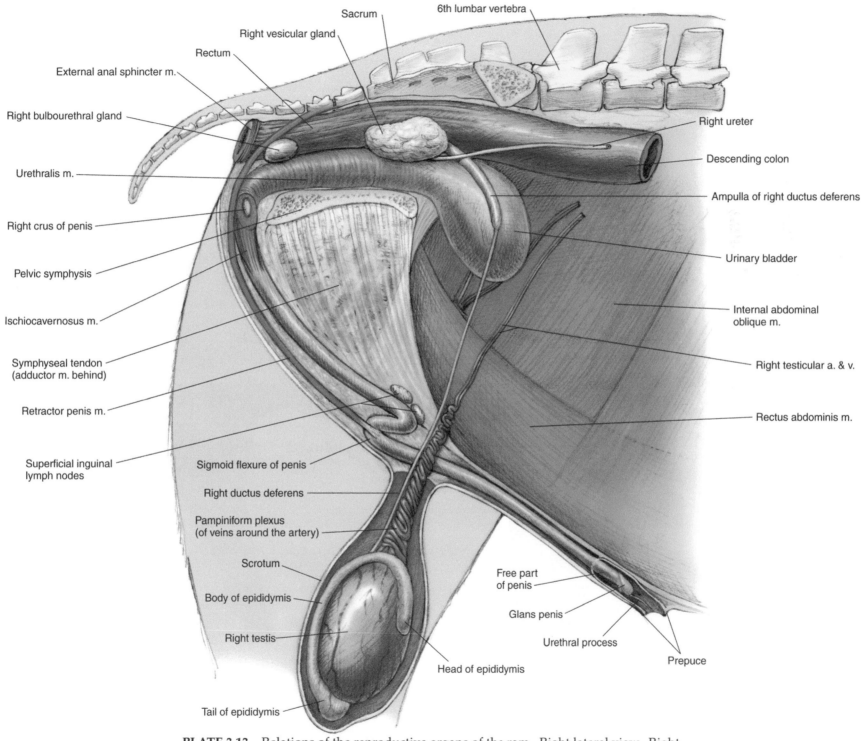

6th lumbar vertebra

Sacrum

Right vesicular gland

Rectum

External anal sphincter m.

Right bulbourethral gland

Urethralis m.

Right crus of penis

Pelvic symphysis

Ischiocavernosus m.

Symphyseal tendon
(adductor m. behind)

Retractor penis m.

Superficial inguinal
lymph nodes

Sigmoid flexure of penis

Right ductus deferens

Pampiniform plexus
(of veins around the artery)

Scrotum

Body of epididymis

Right testis

Tail of epididymis

Head of epididymis

Right ureter

Descending colon

Ampulla of right ductus deferens

Urinary bladder

Internal abdominal
oblique m.

Right testicular a. & v.

Rectus abdominis m.

Free part
of penis

Glans penis

Urethral process

Prepuce

66

PLATE 3.13 Relations of the reproductive organs of the ram. Right lateral view. Right
pelvic limb and body wall are removed. The ram's prostate gland is entirely disseminate;
it lies deep to the urethralis muscle. m = muscle, a = artery, v = vein

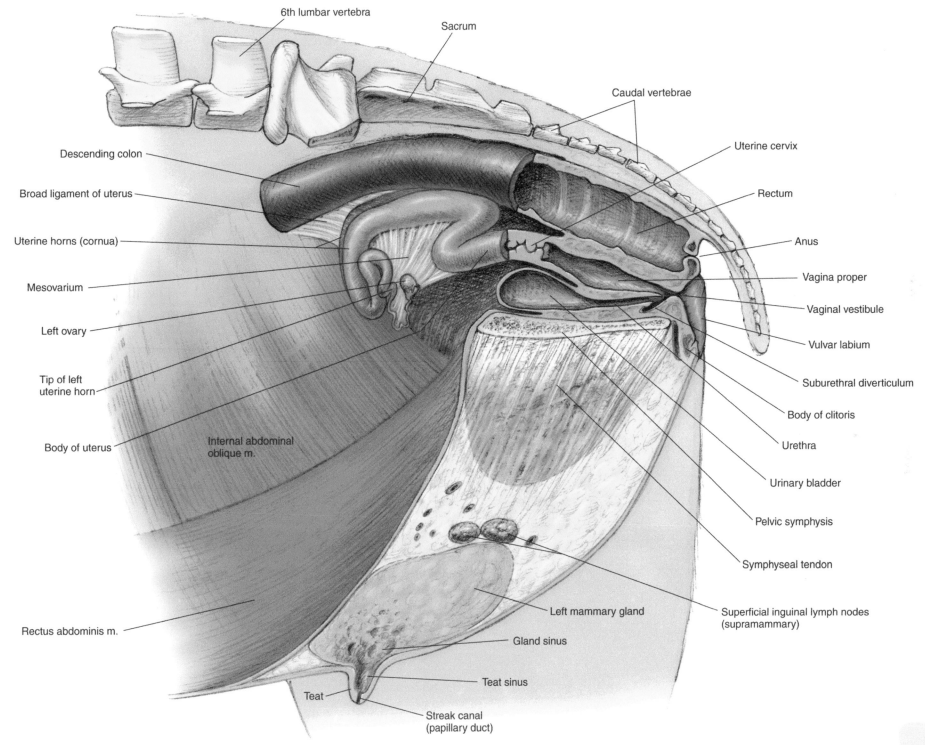

6th lumbar vertebra

Sacrum

Caudal vertebrae

Descending colon

Uterine cervix

Broad ligament of uterus

Rectum

Uterine horns (cornua)

Anus

Mesovarium

Vagina proper

Left ovary

Vaginal vestibule

Tip of left
uterine horn

Vulvar labium

Suburethral diverticulum

Body of uterus

Internal abdominal
oblique m.

Body of clitoris

Urethra

Urinary bladder

Pelvic symphysis

Rectus abdominis m.

Symphyseal tendon

Left mammary gland

Superficial inguinal lymph nodes
(supramammary)

Gland sinus

Teat sinus

Teat

Streak canal
(papillary duct)

PLATE 3.14 Relations of the reproductive organs of the ewe. Left lateral view with partial
median sections of the vagina, uterine cervix, rectum, urinary bladder, and urethra. m = muscle

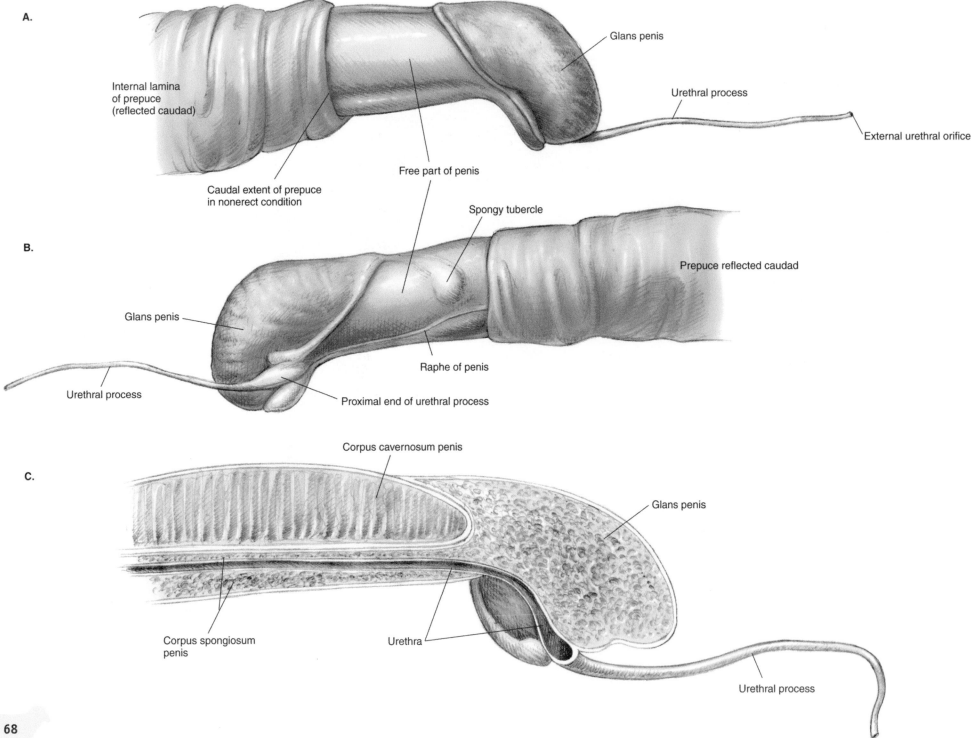

A.

Glans penis

Internal lamina
of prepuce
(reflected caudad)

Urethral process

External urethral orifice

Caudal extent of prepuce
in nonerect condition

Free part of penis

B.

Spongy tubercle

Prepuce reflected caudad

Glans penis

Raphe of penis

Urethral process

Proximal end of urethral process

Corpus cavernosum penis

C.

Glans penis

Corpus spongiosum
penis

Urethra

Urethral process

PLATE 3.15   Penis of the ram. **A.** Cranial portion of the ram's penis. Right lateral view.
B. Left lateral view. **C.** Median section. Right lateral view.

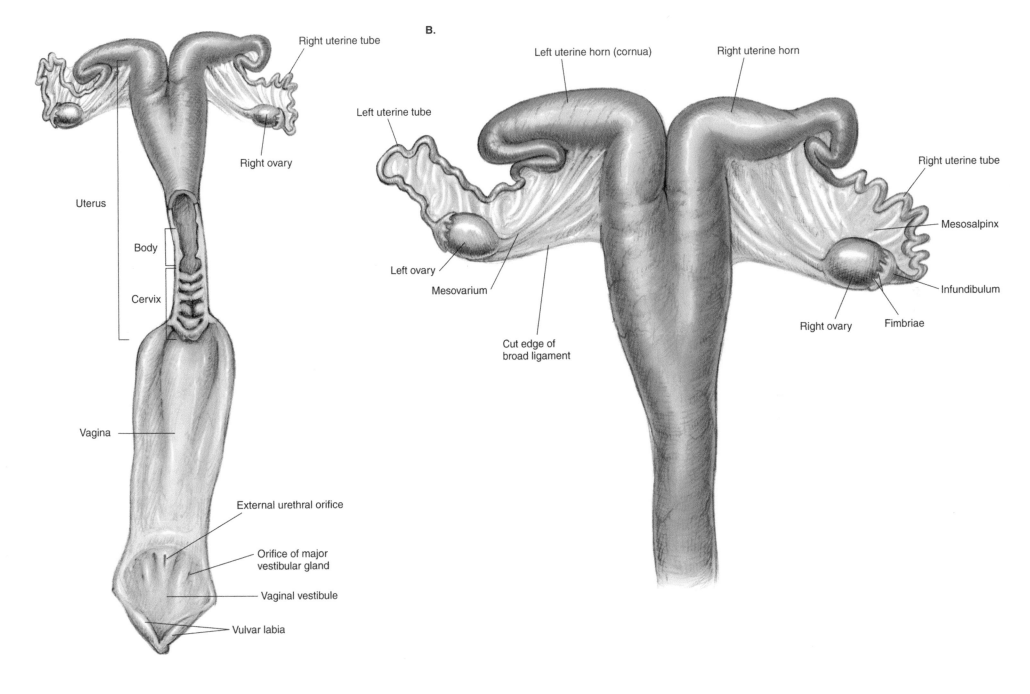

A. Right uterine tube

Right ovary

Uterus

Body

Cervix

Vagina

External urethral orifice

Orifice of major
vestibular gland

Vaginal vestibule

Vulvar labia

B. Left uterine horn (cornua)

Right uterine horn

Left uterine tube

Right uterine tube

Mesosalpinx

Left ovary

Mesovarium

Infundibulum

Cut edge of
broad ligament

Right ovary

Fimbriae

69

PLATE 3.16   **A.** Isolated reproductive organs of the ewe. Vagina and a portion of the uterus
opened dorsally. **B.** Isolated uterus, uterine tubes, and ovaries of the ewe. Dorsal view.

SECTION 4 THE GOAT (*Capra hircus*)

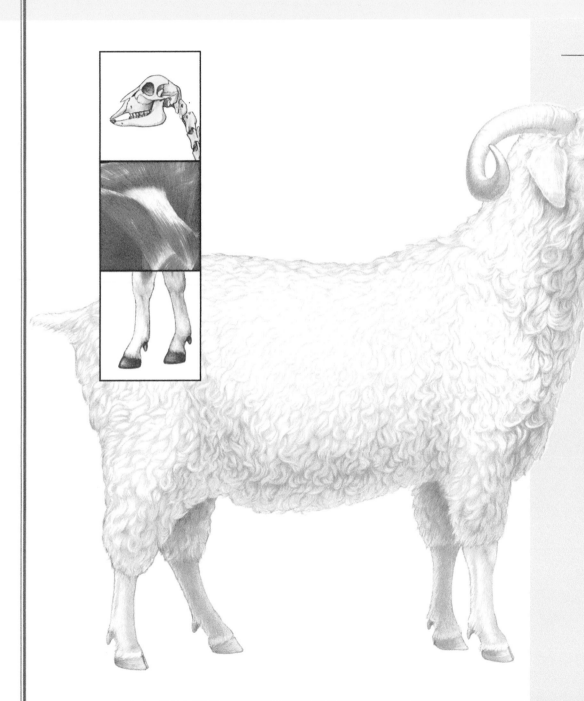

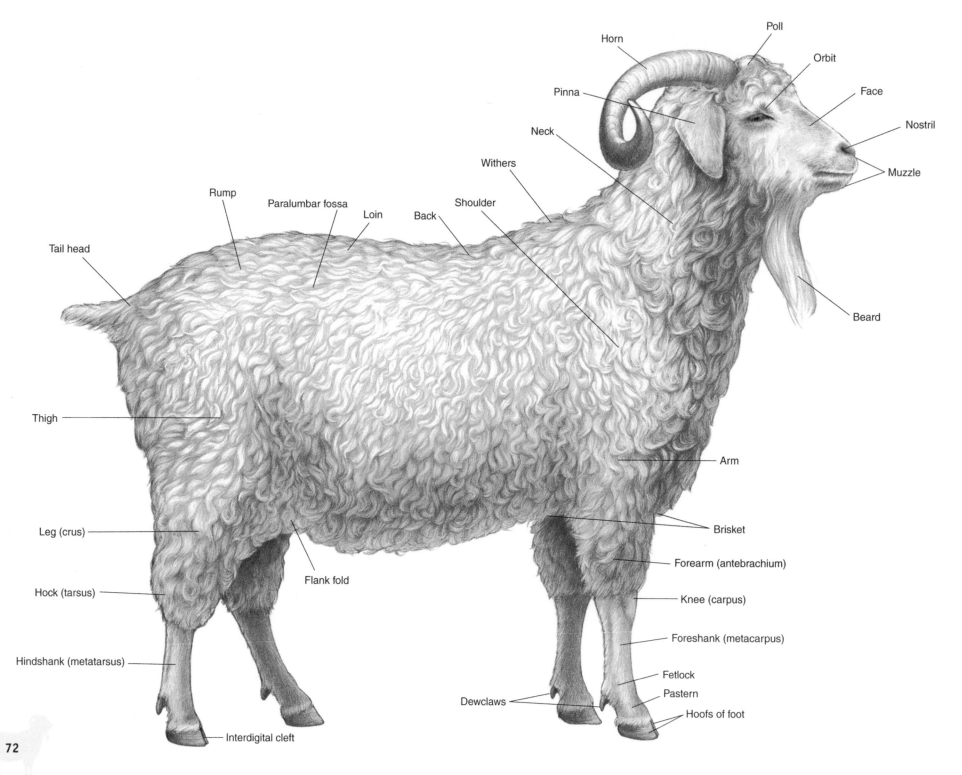

Horn

Poll

Orbit

Pinna

Face

Neck

Nostril

Withers

Muzzle

Rump

Shoulder

Paralumbar fossa

Back

Loin

Tail head

Beard

Thigh

Arm

Brisket

Leg (crus)

Forearm (antebrachium)

Flank fold

Knee (carpus)

Hock (tarsus)

Foreshank (metacarpus)

Hindshank (metatarsus)

Fetlock

Dewclaws

Pastern

Hoofs of foot

Interdigital cleft

72

PLATE 4.1 Right lateral view of an Angora buck (billy).

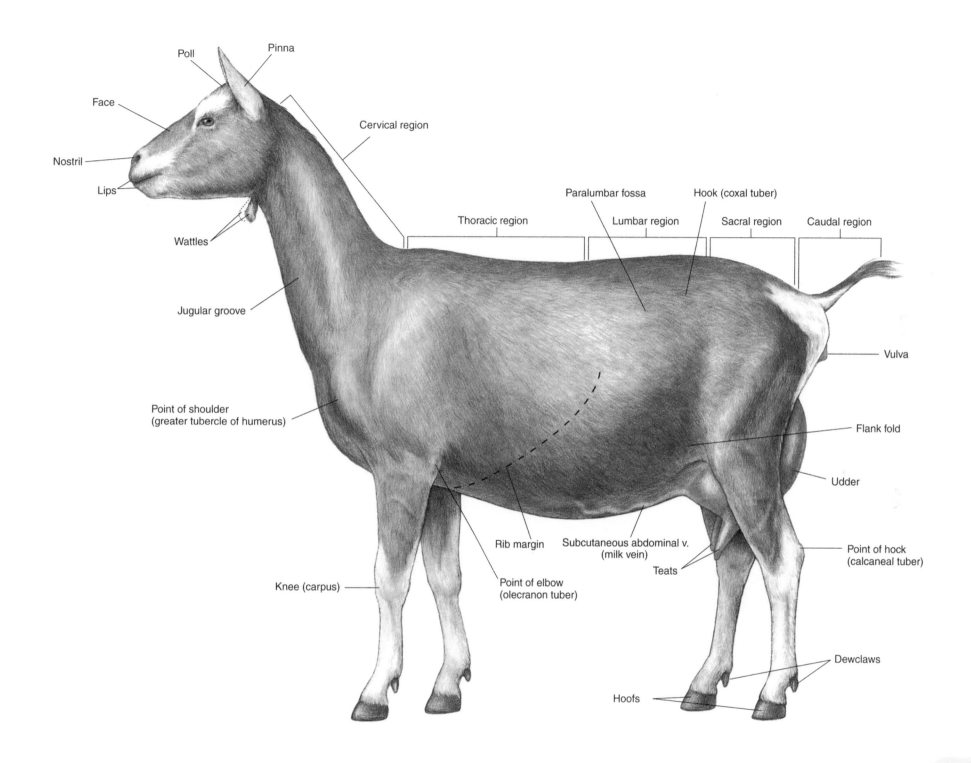

Poll

Pinna

Face

Nostril

Lips

Wattles

Cervical region

Paralumbar fossa

Hook (coxal tuber)

Thoracic region

Lumbar region

Sacral region

Caudal region

Jugular groove

Vulva

Point of shoulder
(greater tubercle of humerus)

Flank fold

Udder

Rib margin

Subcutaneous abdominal v.
(milk vein)

Point of hock
(calcaneal tuber)

Teats

Knee (carpus)

Point of elbow
(olecranon tuber)

Dewclaws

Hoofs

73

PLATE 4.2 Left lateral view of a Toggenberg doe (nanny).
Dorsal vertebral regions are indicated. v = vein

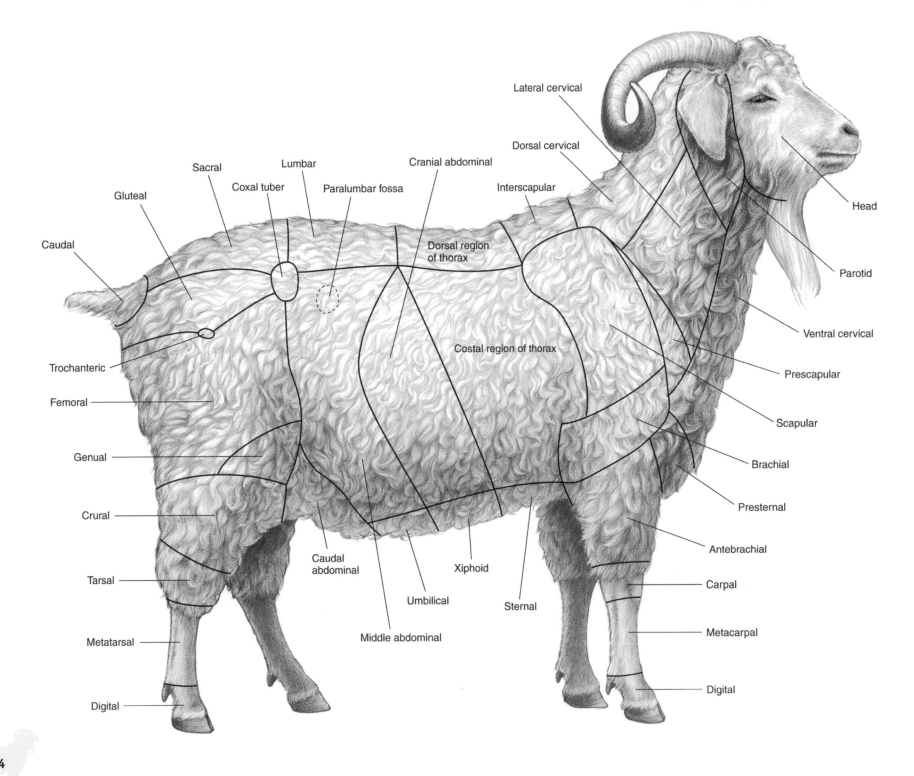

Lateral cervical

Dorsal cervical

Sacral

Lumbar

Cranial abdominal

Coxal tuber

Paralumbar fossa

Interscapular

Gluteal

Head

Caudal

Dorsal region
of thorax

Parotid

Trochanteric

Costal region of thorax

Ventral cervical

Femoral

Prescapular

Genual

Scapular

Brachial

Crural

Presternal

Tarsal

Caudal
abdominal

Xiphoid

Antebrachial

Metatarsal

Umbilical

Sternal

Carpal

Digital

Middle abdominal

Metacarpal

Digital

PLATE 4.3   Body regions of the goat. Right lateral view.

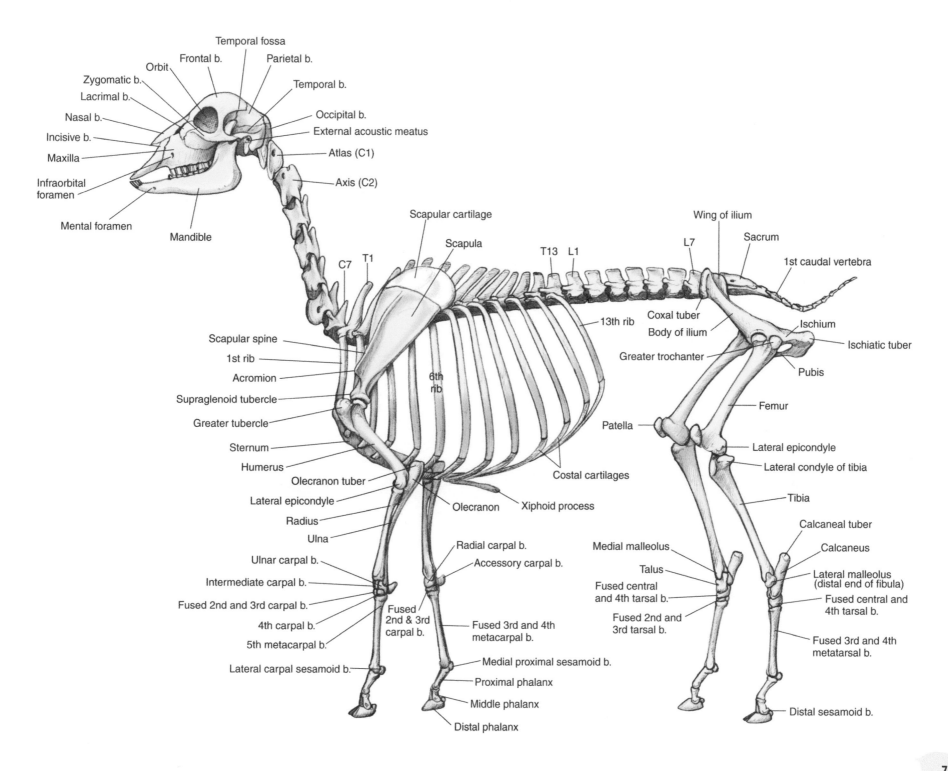

Temporal fossa

Frontal b.

Orbit

Zygomatic b.

Lacrimal b.

Nasal b.

Incisive b.

Maxilla

Infraorbital foramen

Mental foramen

Mandible

Parietal b.

Temporal b.

Occipital b.

External acoustic meatus

Atlas (C1)

Axis (C2)

Scapular cartilage

Scapula

C7 T1

Scapular spine

1st rib

Acromion

Supraglenoid tubercle

Greater tubercle

Sternum

Humerus

Olecranon tuber

Lateral epicondyle

Radius

Ulna

Ulnar carpal b.

Intermediate carpal b.

Fused 2nd and 3rd carpal b.

4th carpal b.

5th metacarpal b.

Lateral carpal sesamoid b.

6th rib

Radial carpal b.

Accessory carpal b.

Fused 2nd & 3rd carpal b.

Fused 3rd and 4th metacarpal b.

Medial proximal sesamoid b.

Proximal phalanx

Middle phalanx

Distal phalanx

Olecranon

Xiphoid process

Costal cartilages

T13 L1

13th rib

L7

Wing of ilium

Sacrum

1st caudal vertebra

Coxal tuber

Body of ilium

Greater trochanter

Patella

Ischium

Ischiatic tuber

Pubis

Femur

Lateral epicondyle

Lateral condyle of tibia

Tibia

Calcaneal tuber

Calcaneus

Lateral malleolus (distal end of fibula)

Fused central and 4th tarsal b.

Fused 3rd and 4th metatarsal b.

Medial malleolus

Talus

Fused central and 4th tarsal b.

Fused 2nd and 3rd tarsal b.

Distal sesamoid b.

PLATE 4.4 Skeleton of the goat. Left lateral view. b = bone, C = cervical vertebra, T = thoracic vertebra, L = lumbar vertebra

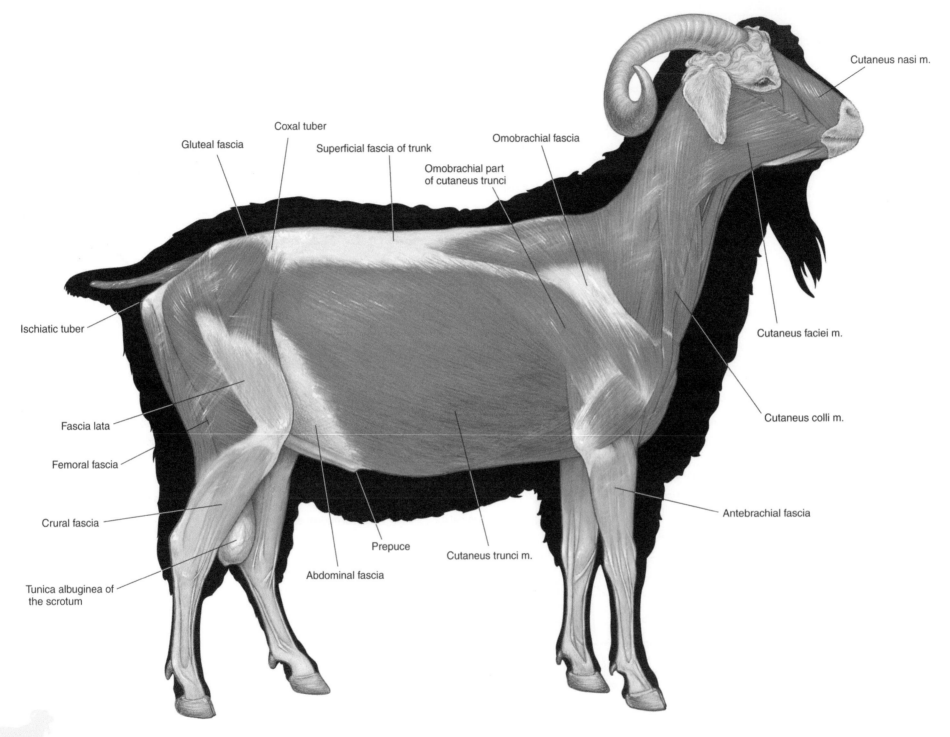

Cutaneus nasi m.

Coxal tuber

Gluteal fascia

Superficial fascia of trunk

Omobrachial fascia

Omobrachial part
of cutaneus trunci

Ischiatic tuber

Cutaneus faciei m.

Fascia lata

Cutaneus colli m.

Femoral fascia

Crural fascia

Antebrachial fascia

Prepuce

Cutaneus trunci m.

Abdominal fascia

Tunica albuginea of
the scrotum

76

PLATE 4.5 Cutaneous muscles and major fasciae of the buck. Right lateral view. m = muscle

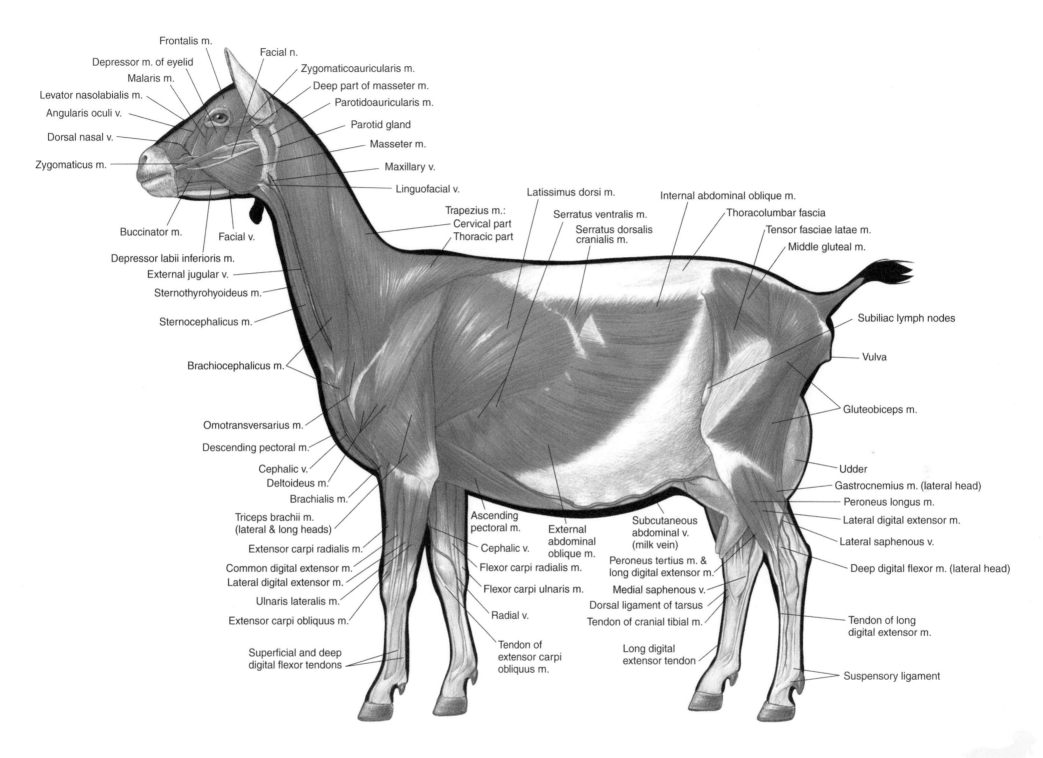

Frontalis m.
Depressor m. of eyelid
Malaris m.
Levator nasolabialis m.
Angularis oculi v.
Dorsal nasal v.
Zygomaticus m.
Buccinator m.
Depressor labii inferioris m.
External jugular v.
Sternothyrohyoideus m.
Sternocephalicus m.
Brachiocephalicus m.
Omotransversarius m.
Descending pectoral m.
Cephalic v.
Deltoideus m.
Brachialis m.
Triceps brachii m.
(lateral & long heads)
Extensor carpi radialis m.
Common digital extensor m.
Lateral digital extensor m.
Ulnaris lateralis m.
Extensor carpi obliquus m.
Superficial and deep
digital flexor tendons

Facial n.
Zygomaticoauricularis m.
Deep part of masseter m.
Parotidoauricularis m.
Parotid gland
Masseter m.
Maxillary v.
Linguofacial v.

Facial v.

Ascending
pectoral m.
Cephalic v.
Flexor carpi radialis m.
Flexor carpi ulnaris m.
Radial v.
Tendon of
extensor carpi
obliquus m.

Latissimus dorsi m.

Trapezius m.:
Cervical part
Thoracic part

Serratus ventralis m.
Serratus dorsalis
cranialis m.

External
abdominal
oblique m.

Subcutaneous
abdominal v.
(milk vein)
Peroneus tertius m. &
long digital extensor m.
Medial saphenous v.
Dorsal ligament of tarsus
Tendon of cranial tibial m.

Long digital
extensor tendon

Internal abdominal oblique m.
Thoracolumbar fascia
Tensor fasciae latae m.
Middle gluteal m.

Subiliac lymph nodes

Vulva

Gluteobiceps m.

Udder
Gastrocnemius m. (lateral head)
Peroneus longus m.
Lateral digital extensor m.
Lateral saphenous v.

Deep digital flexor m. (lateral head)

Tendon of long
digital extensor m.

Suspensory ligament

77

PLATE 4.6 Superficial muscles and veins of the doe. Left lateral view. m = muscle, v = vein

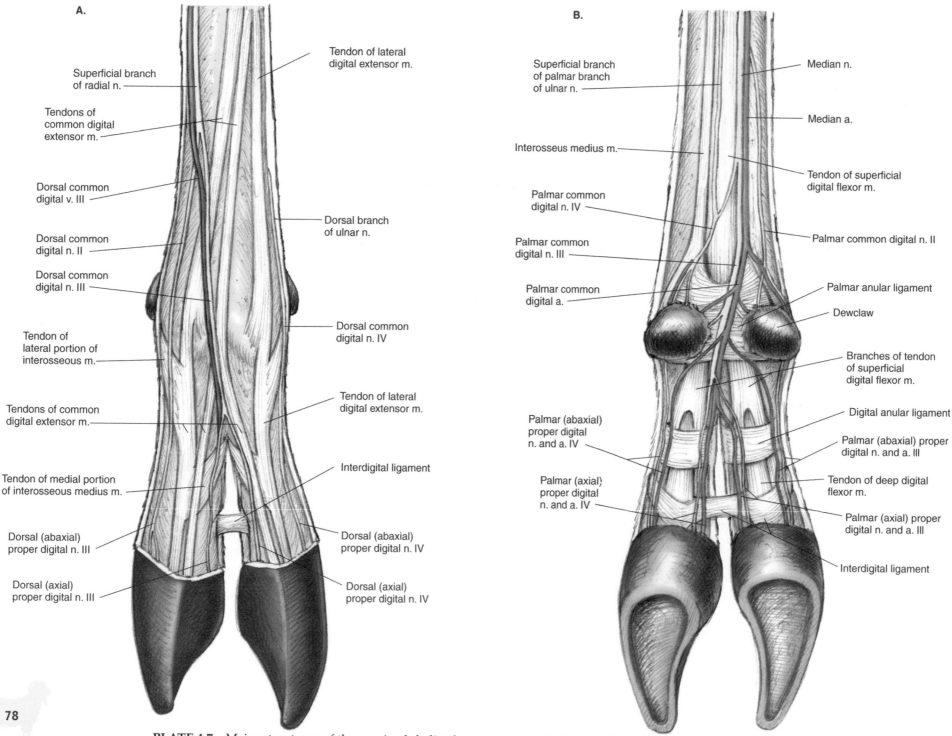

A.

Superficial branch of radial n.

Tendons of common digital extensor m.

Dorsal common digital v. III

Dorsal common digital n. II

Dorsal common digital n. III

Tendon of lateral portion of interosseous m.

Tendons of common digital extensor m.

Tendon of medial portion of interosseous medius m.

Dorsal (abaxial) proper digital n. III

Dorsal (axial) proper digital n. III

Tendon of lateral digital extensor m.

Dorsal branch of ulnar n.

Dorsal common digital n. IV

Tendon of lateral digital extensor m.

Interdigital ligament

Dorsal (abaxial) proper digital n. IV

Dorsal (axial) proper digital n. IV

B.

Superficial branch of palmar branch of ulnar n.

Interosseus medius m.

Palmar common digital n. IV

Palmar common digital n. III

Palmar common digital a.

Palmar (abaxial) proper digital n. and a. IV

Palmar (axial) proper digital n. and a. IV

Median n.

Median a.

Tendon of superficial digital flexor m.

Palmar common digital n. II

Palmar anular ligament

Dewclaw

Branches of tendon of superficial digital flexor m.

Digital anular ligament

Palmar (abaxial) proper digital n. and a. III

Tendon of deep digital flexor m.

Palmar (axial) proper digital n. and a. III

Interdigital ligament

PLATE 4.7   Major structures of the caprine left distal metacarpus and digits. **A.** Dorsal view, arteries excluded. **B.** Palmar view, veins excluded. n = nerve, m = muscle, a = artery

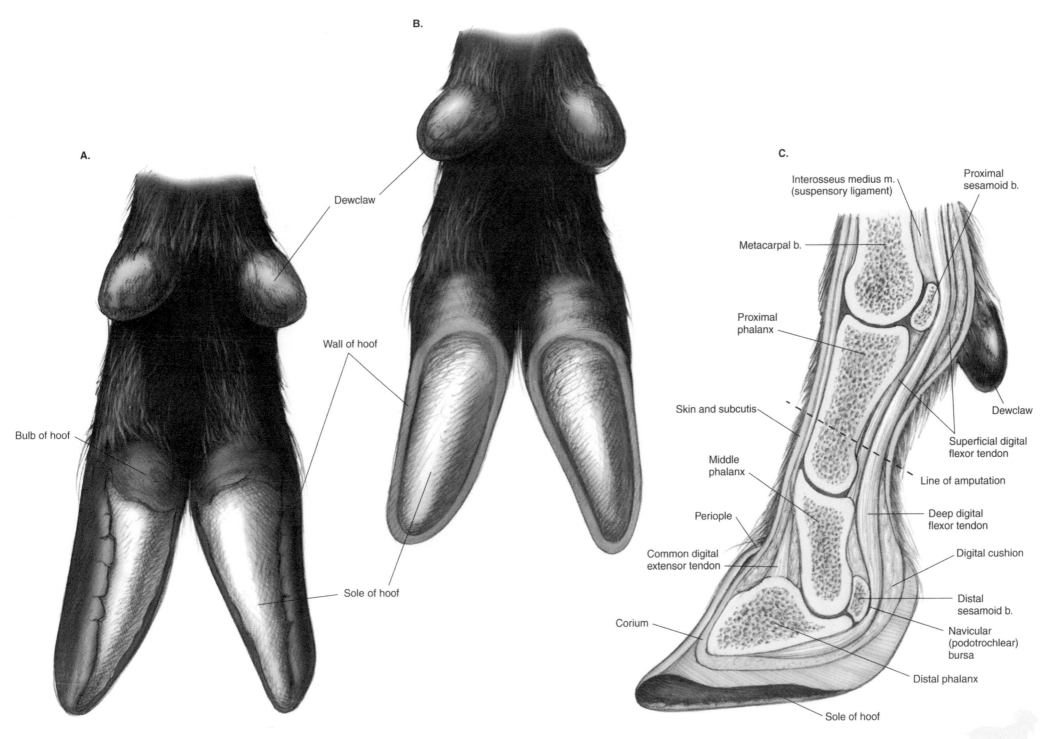

A.

Dewclaw

Wall of hoof

Bulb of hoof

Sole of hoof

B.

C.

Interosseus medius m. (suspensory ligament)

Proximal sesamoid b.

Metacarpal b.

Proximal phalanx

Skin and subcutis

Dewclaw

Superficial digital flexor tendon

Line of amputation

Middle phalanx

Periople

Deep digital flexor tendon

Common digital extensor tendon

Digital cushion

Corium

Distal sesamoid b.

Navicular (podotrochlear) bursa

Distal phalanx

Sole of hoof

PLATE 4.8 **A.** Untrimmed hoofs of the goat. **B.** Trimmed hoofs of the goat. **C.** Parasagittal section through the fetlock and digit. For artiodactyls, claw is synonymous with hoof. When kept on soft ground, a mature goat's hoofs should be trimmed every 4–5 months. b = bone

79

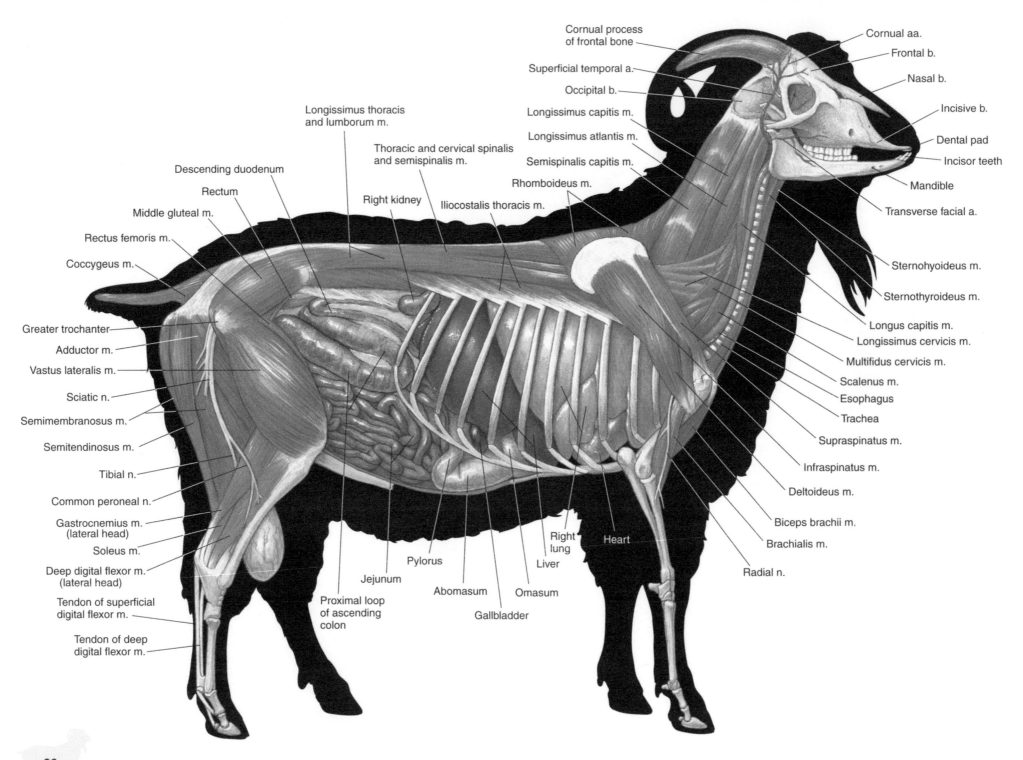

Cornual process
of frontal bone

Superficial temporal a.

Occipital b.

Longissimus thoracis
and lumborum m.

Thoracic and cervical spinalis
and semispinalis m.

Descending duodenum

Rectum

Right kidney

Middle gluteal m.

Longissimus capitis m.

Longissimus atlantis m.

Semispinalis capitis m.

Rhomboideus m.

Iliocostalis thoracis m.

Cornual aa.

Frontal b.

Nasal b.

Incisive b.

Dental pad

Incisor teeth

Mandible

Transverse facial a.

Rectus femoris m.

Coccygeus m.

Greater trochanter

Adductor m.

Vastus lateralis m.

Sciatic n.

Semimembranosus m.

Semitendinosus m.

Tibial n.

Common peroneal n.

Gastrocnemius m.
(lateral head)

Soleus m.

Deep digital flexor m.
(lateral head)

Tendon of superficial
digital flexor m.

Tendon of deep
digital flexor m.

Proximal loop
of ascending
colon

Jejunum

Pylorus

Abomasum

Gallbladder

Omasum

Liver

Right
lung

Heart

Sternohyoideus m.

Sternothyroideus m.

Longus capitis m.

Longissimus cervicis m.

Multifidus cervicis m.

Scalenus m.

Esophagus

Trachea

Supraspinatus m.

Infraspinatus m.

Deltoideus m.

Biceps brachii m.

Brachialis m.

Radial n.

80

PLATE 4.9   Deep muscles and *in situ* viscera of the buck. Greater omentum is removed.
Right lateral view. m = muscle, n = nerve, a = artery, b = bone

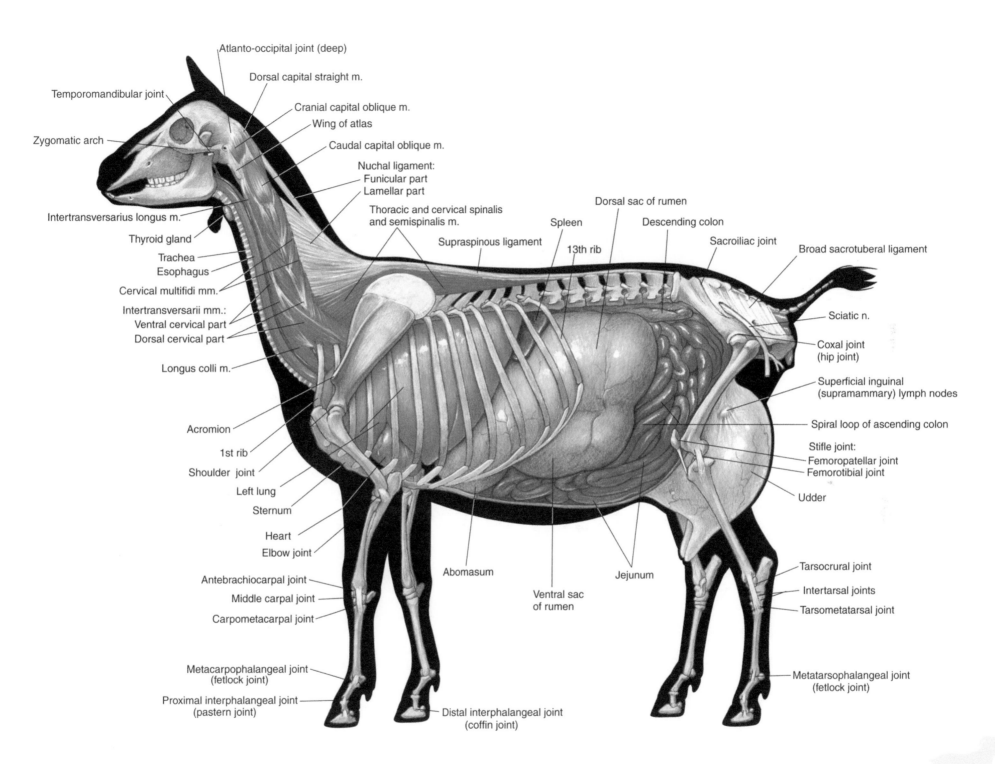

Atlanto-occipital joint (deep)

Dorsal capital straight m.

Temporomandibular joint

Cranial capital oblique m.

Wing of atlas

Zygomatic arch

Caudal capital oblique m.

Nuchal ligament:
Funicular part
Lamellar part

Thoracic and cervical spinalis
and semispinalis m.

Dorsal sac of rumen

Intertransversarius longus m.

Spleen

Descending colon

Supraspinous ligament

Sacroiliac joint

Thyroid gland

13th rib

Broad sacrotuberal ligament

Trachea

Esophagus

Cervical multifidi mm.

Intertransversarii mm.:
Ventral cervical part
Dorsal cervical part

Sciatic n.

Coxal joint
(hip joint)

Longus colli m.

Superficial inguinal
(supramammary) lymph nodes

Acromion

Spiral loop of ascending colon

1st rib

Stifle joint:
Femoropatellar joint
Femorotibial joint

Shoulder joint

Left lung

Sternum

Udder

Heart

Elbow joint

Tarsocrural joint

Antebrachiocarpal joint

Intertarsal joints

Middle carpal joint

Abomasum

Jejunum

Tarsometatarsal joint

Carpometacarpal joint

Ventral sac
of rumen

Metacarpophalangeal joint
(fetlock joint)

Metatarsophalangeal joint
(fetlock joint)

Proximal interphalangeal joint
(pastern joint)

Distal interphalangeal joint
(coffin joint)

81

PLATE 4.10 Deep cervical muscles, *in situ* viscera, skeleton, and major joints of the doe.
Left lateral view. m = muscle, n = nerve

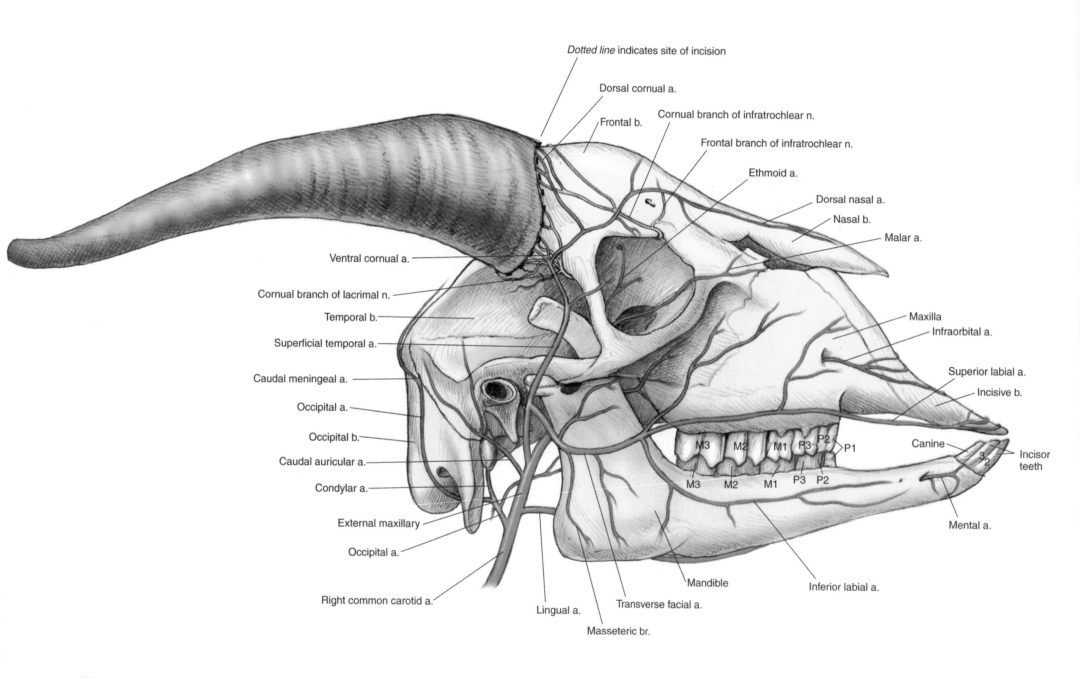

Dotted line indicates site of incision

Dorsal cornual a.

Frontal b.

Cornual branch of infratrochlear n.

Frontal branch of infratrochlear n.

Ethmoid a.

Dorsal nasal a.

Nasal b.

Malar a.

Ventral cornual a.

Cornual branch of lacrimal n.

Temporal b.

Maxilla

Superficial temporal a.

Infraorbital a.

Caudal meningeal a.

Superior labial a.

Occipital a.

Incisive b.

Occipital b.

M3 M2 M1 P3 P2 P1

Canine

Caudal auricular a.

Incisor teeth

$\frac{3}{2}$

Condylar a.

M3 M2 M1 P3 P2

Mental a.

External maxillary

Occipital a.

Right common carotid a.

Lingual a.

Transverse facial a.

Masseteric br.

Mandible

Inferior labial a.

PLATE 4.11   Superficial structures of the goat's head.   *Dashed line* indicates the site of a dehorning incision.
a = artery, b = bone, n = nerve, M = molar tooth, P = premolar tooth

82

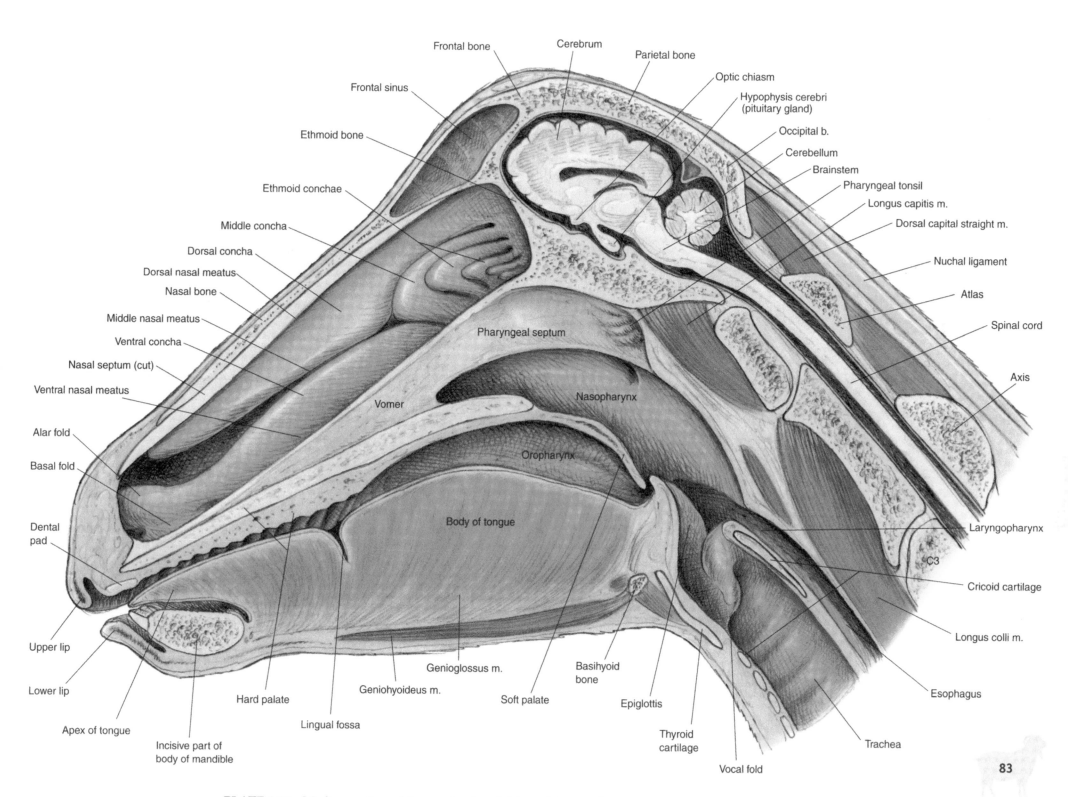

Frontal bone
Cerebrum
Parietal bone
Frontal sinus
Optic chiasm
Hypophysis cerebri
(pituitary gland)
Ethmoid bone
Occipital b.
Cerebellum
Ethmoid conchae
Brainstem
Pharyngeal tonsil
Middle concha
Longus capitis m.
Dorsal concha
Dorsal nasal meatus
Dorsal capital straight m.
Nasal bone
Nuchal ligament
Middle nasal meatus
Pharyngeal septum
Atlas
Ventral concha
Spinal cord
Nasal septum (cut)
Nasopharynx
Ventral nasal meatus
Axis
Vomer
Alar fold
Oropharynx
Basal fold
Body of tongue
Laryngopharynx
Dental
pad
C3
Cricoid cartilage
Upper lip
Longus colli m.
Lower lip
Genioglossus m.
Basihyoid
bone
Esophagus
Apex of tongue
Geniohyoideus m.
Soft palate
Epiglottis
Incisive part of
body of mandible
Hard palate
Trachea
Lingual fossa
Thyroid
cartilage
Vocal fold

PLATE 4.12   Median section of the caprine head. Most of the nasal septum is removed. m = muscle, b = bone

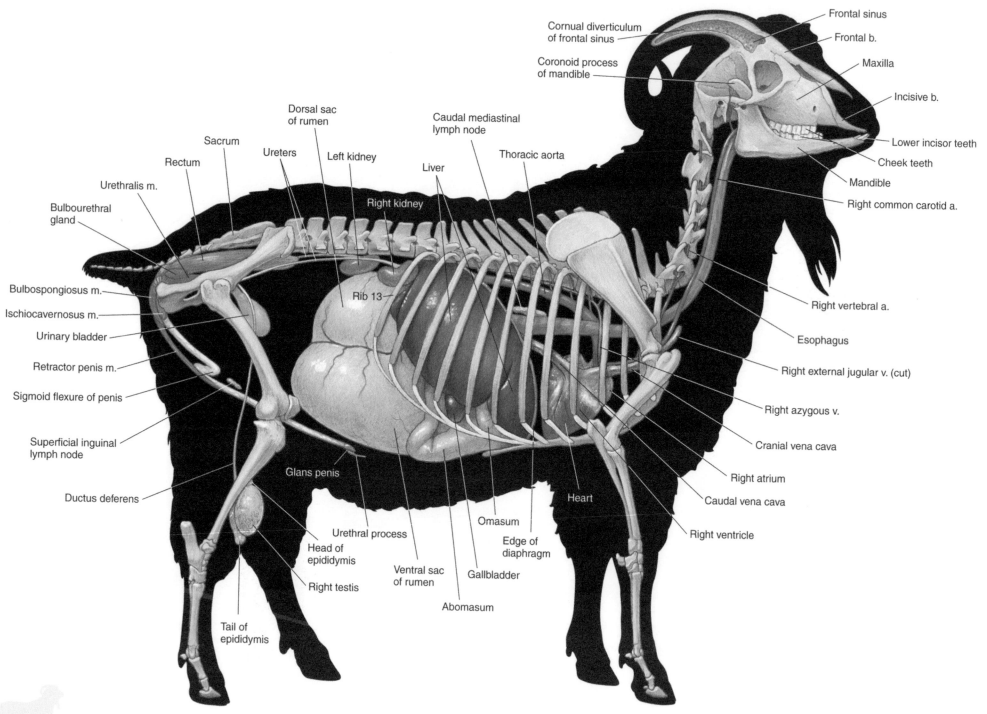

Cornual diverticulum of frontal sinus

Frontal sinus

Frontal b.

Coronoid process of mandible

Maxilla

Incisive b.

Dorsal sac of rumen

Caudal mediastinal lymph node

Sacrum

Ureters

Left kidney

Liver

Thoracic aorta

Lower incisor teeth

Cheek teeth

Rectum

Right kidney

Mandible

Urethralis m.

Right common carotid a.

Bulbourethral gland

Rib 13

Bulbospongiosus m.

Right vertebral a.

Ischiocavernosus m.

Esophagus

Urinary bladder

Retractor penis m.

Right external jugular v. (cut)

Sigmoid flexure of penis

Right azygous v.

Cranial vena cava

Superficial inguinal lymph node

Glans penis

Right atrium

Ductus deferens

Heart

Caudal vena cava

Urethral process

Omasum

Right ventricle

Head of epididymis

Edge of diaphragm

Right testis

Ventral sac of rumen

Gallbladder

Tail of epididymis

Abomasum

84

PLATE 4.13 Reproductive organs, abdominal viscera, heart, and adjacent major vessels related to the skeleton of the buck. Intestines and lungs removed. Right lateral view.
m = muscle, v = vein, a = artery, b = bone

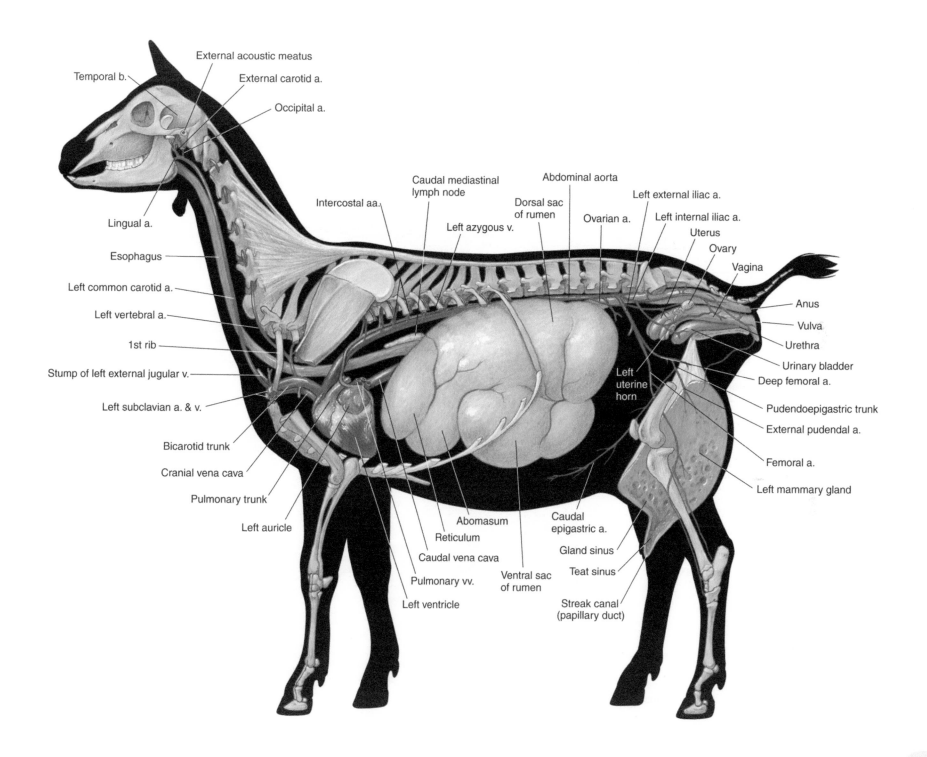

Temporal b.
External acoustic meatus
External carotid a.
Occipital a.
Lingual a.
Esophagus
Left common carotid a.
Left vertebral a.
1st rib
Stump of left external jugular v.
Left subclavian a. & v.
Bicarotid trunk
Cranial vena cava
Pulmonary trunk
Left auricle
Left ventricle
Pulmonary vv.
Caudal vena cava
Reticulum
Abomasum
Ventral sac of rumen
Caudal mediastinal lymph node
Intercostal aa.
Left azygous v.
Dorsal sac of rumen
Abdominal aorta
Ovarian a.
Left external iliac a.
Left internal iliac a.
Uterus
Ovary
Vagina
Anus
Vulva
Urethra
Urinary bladder
Left uterine horn
Deep femoral a.
Pudendoepigastric trunk
External pudendal a.
Femoral a.
Left mammary gland
Caudal epigastric a.
Gland sinus
Teat sinus
Streak canal (papillary duct)

PLATE 4.14 Reproductive organs, abdominal viscera, heart, and adjacent major vessels of the doe. Ribs 2 and 12 and the lungs and intestines are removed. Left lateral view. a = artery, b = bone, v = vein

85

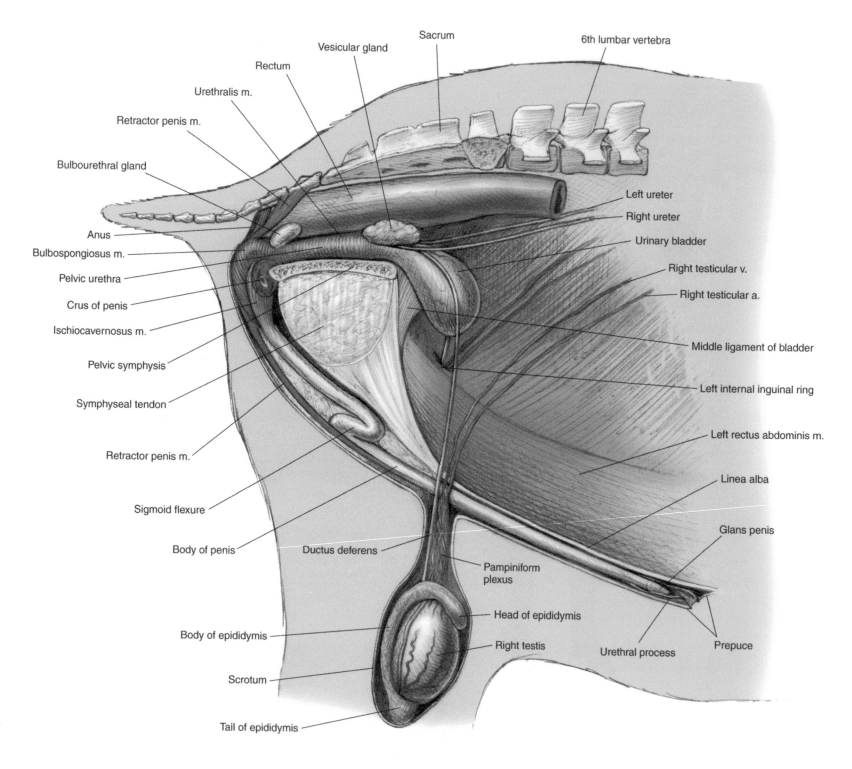

Sacrum

Vesicular gland

6th lumbar vertebra

Rectum

Urethralis m.

Retractor penis m.

Bulbourethral gland

Left ureter

Right ureter

Anus

Urinary bladder

Bulbospongiosus m.

Right testicular v.

Pelvic urethra

Right testicular a.

Crus of penis

Ischiocavernosus m.

Middle ligament of bladder

Pelvic symphysis

Left internal inguinal ring

Symphyseal tendon

Left rectus abdominis m.

Retractor penis m.

Linea alba

Sigmoid flexure

Glans penis

Body of penis

Ductus deferens

Pampiniform plexus

Head of epididymis

Body of epididymis

Prepuce

Right testis

Urethral process

Scrotum

Tail of epididymis

86

PLATE 4.15 Relations of the reproductive organs of the buck. Right pelvic limb and body wall are removed. Right lateral view. a = artery, m = muscle, v = vein

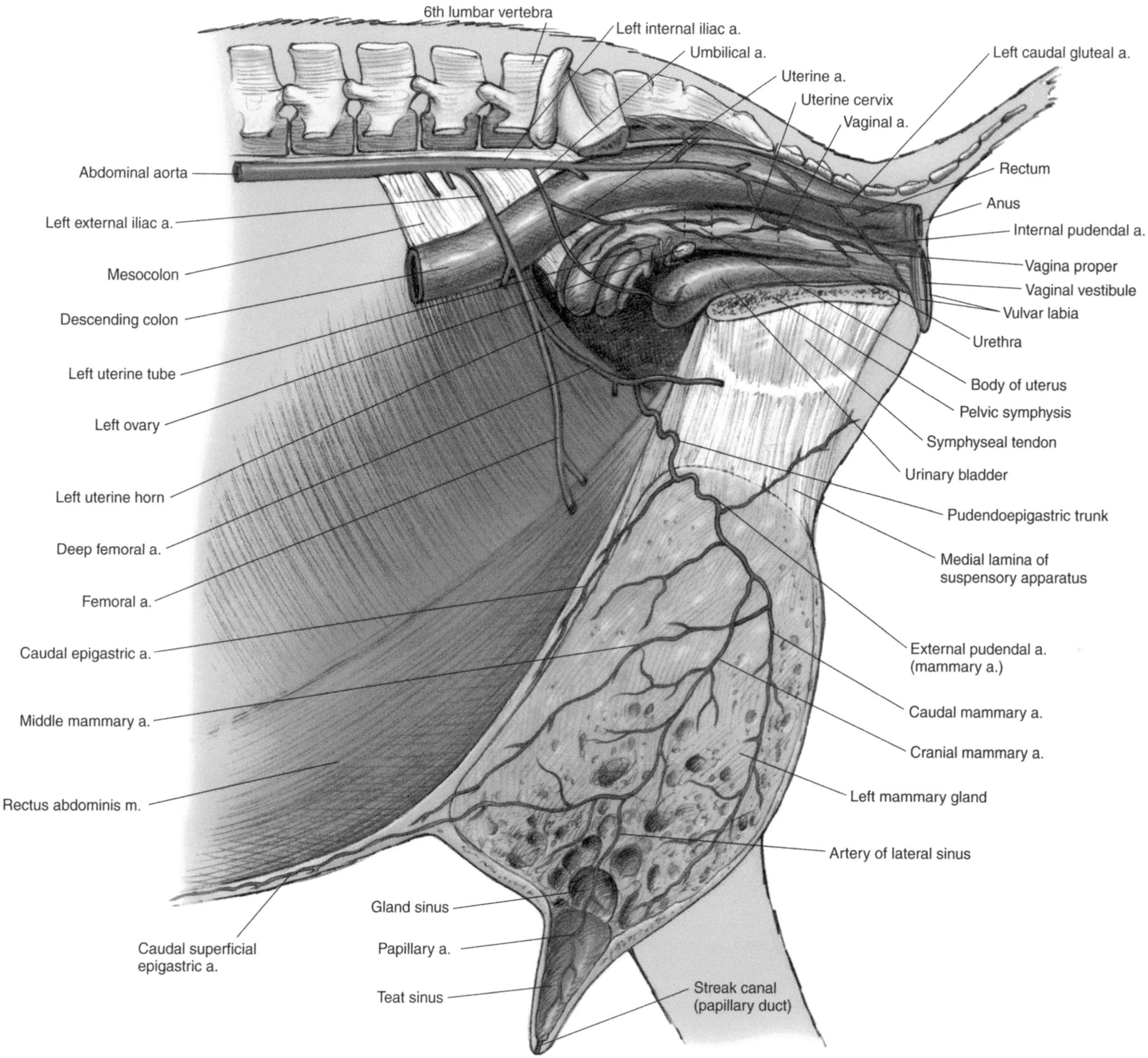

6th lumbar vertebra

Left internal iliac a.

Umbilical a.

Uterine a.

Uterine cervix

Vaginal a.

Left caudal gluteal a.

Rectum

Anus

Internal pudendal a.

Vagina proper

Vaginal vestibule

Vulvar labia

Urethra

Body of uterus

Pelvic symphysis

Symphyseal tendon

Urinary bladder

Pudendoepigastric trunk

Medial lamina of suspensory apparatus

External pudendal a. (mammary a.)

Caudal mammary a.

Cranial mammary a.

Left mammary gland

Artery of lateral sinus

Abdominal aorta

Left external iliac a.

Mesocolon

Descending colon

Left uterine tube

Left ovary

Left uterine horn

Deep femoral a.

Femoral a.

Caudal epigastric a.

Middle mammary a.

Rectus abdominis m.

Caudal superficial epigastric a.

Gland sinus

Papillary a.

Teat sinus

Streak canal (papillary duct)

PLATE 4.16   Relations of the reproductive organs of the doe.
Median section. a = artery, m = muscle

SECTION 5 THE LLAMA AND ALPACA
(*Lama glama* and *Lama pacos*)

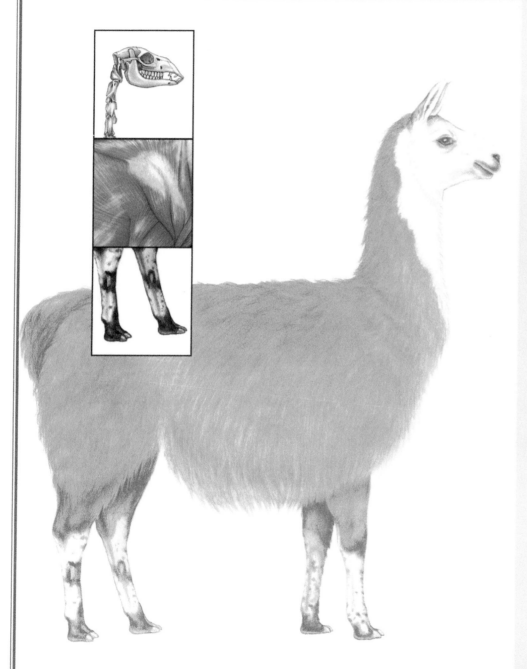

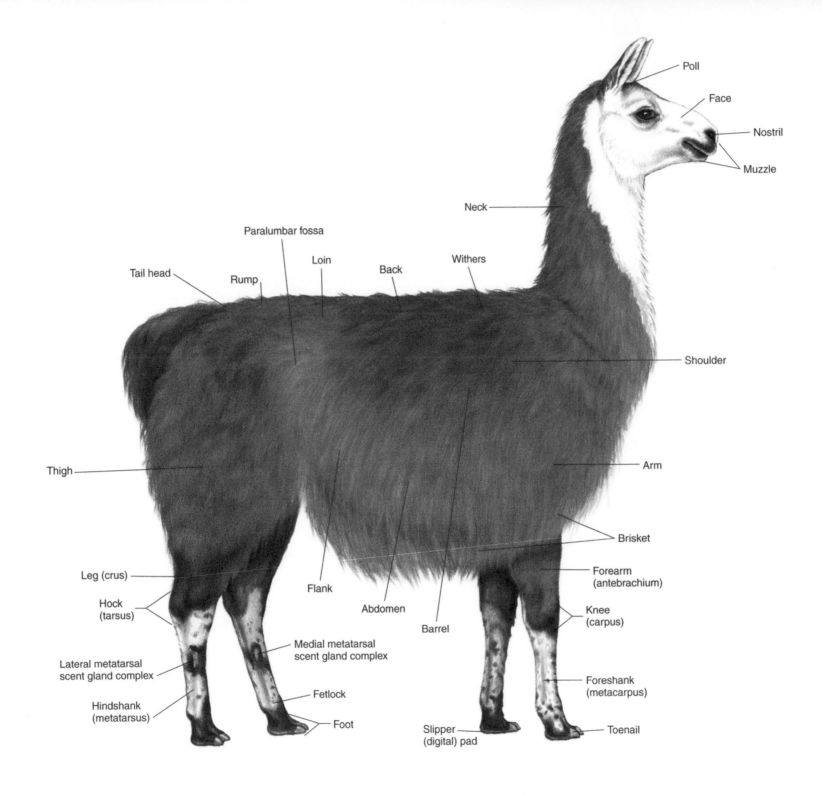

PLATE 5.1 Right lateral view of a male llama.

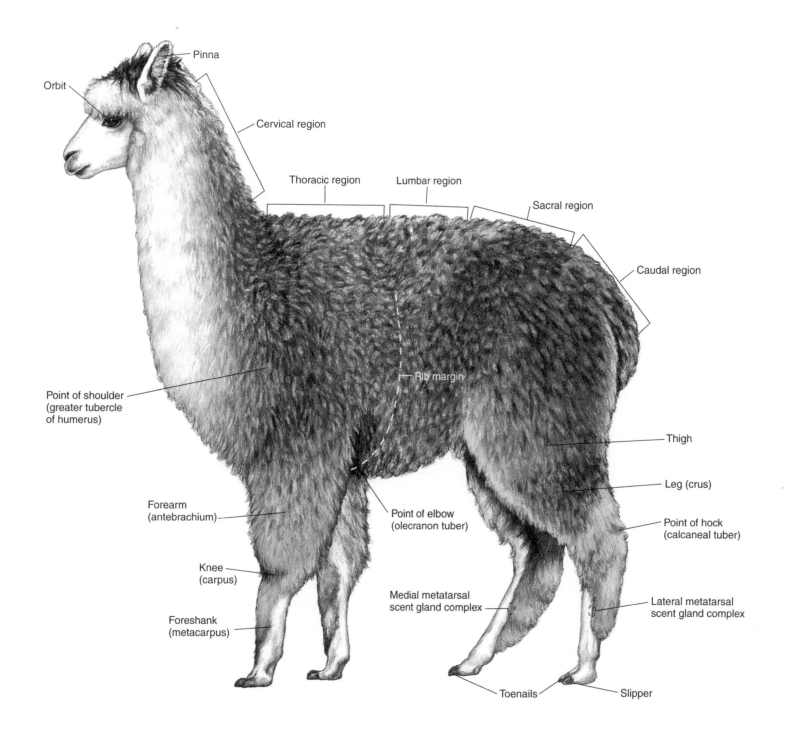

Orbit

Pinna

Cervical region

Thoracic region

Lumbar region

Sacral region

Caudal region

Rib margin

Point of shoulder
(greater tubercle
of humerus)

Thigh

Leg (crus)

Forearm
(antebrachium)

Point of elbow
(olecranon tuber)

Point of hock
(calcaneal tuber)

Knee
(carpus)

Medial metatarsal
scent gland complex

Lateral metatarsal
scent gland complex

Foreshank
(metacarpus)

Toenails

Slipper

PLATE 5.2   Left lateral view of a female huacaya alpaca. Dorsal vertebral regions are indicated.

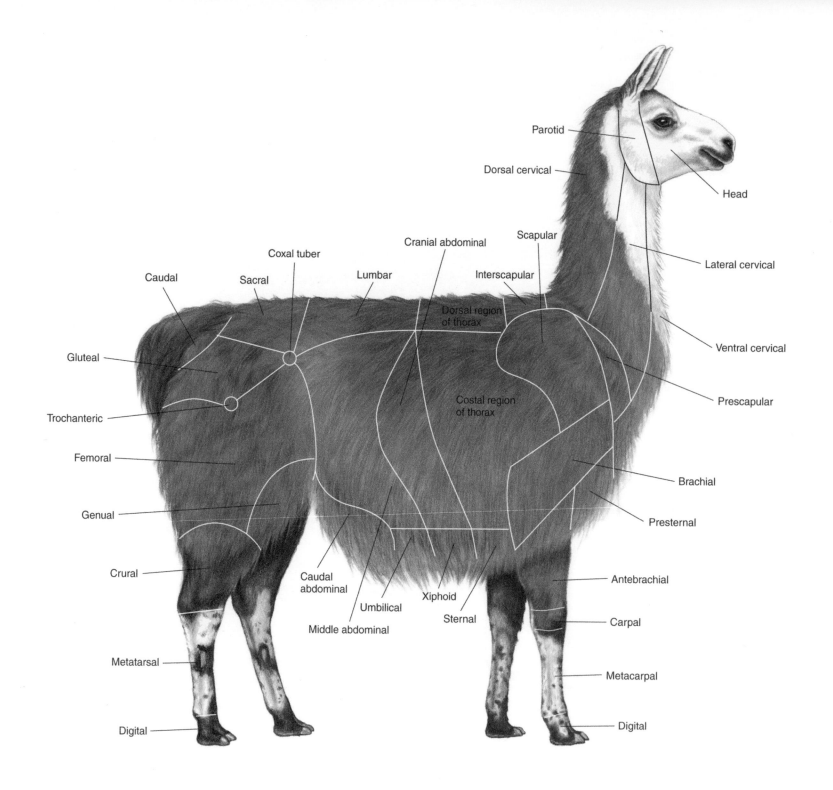

Parotid

Dorsal cervical

Head

Scapular

Cranial abdominal

Lateral cervical

Coxal tuber

Interscapular

Caudal

Sacral

Lumbar

Dorsal region
of thorax

Gluteal

Ventral cervical

Costal region
of thorax

Prescapular

Trochanteric

Femoral

Brachial

Genual

Presternal

Crural

Antebrachial

Caudal
abdominal

Xiphoid

Carpal

Umbilical

Sternal

Middle abdominal

Metatarsal

Metacarpal

Digital

Digital

PLATE 5.3 Body regions of the llama.

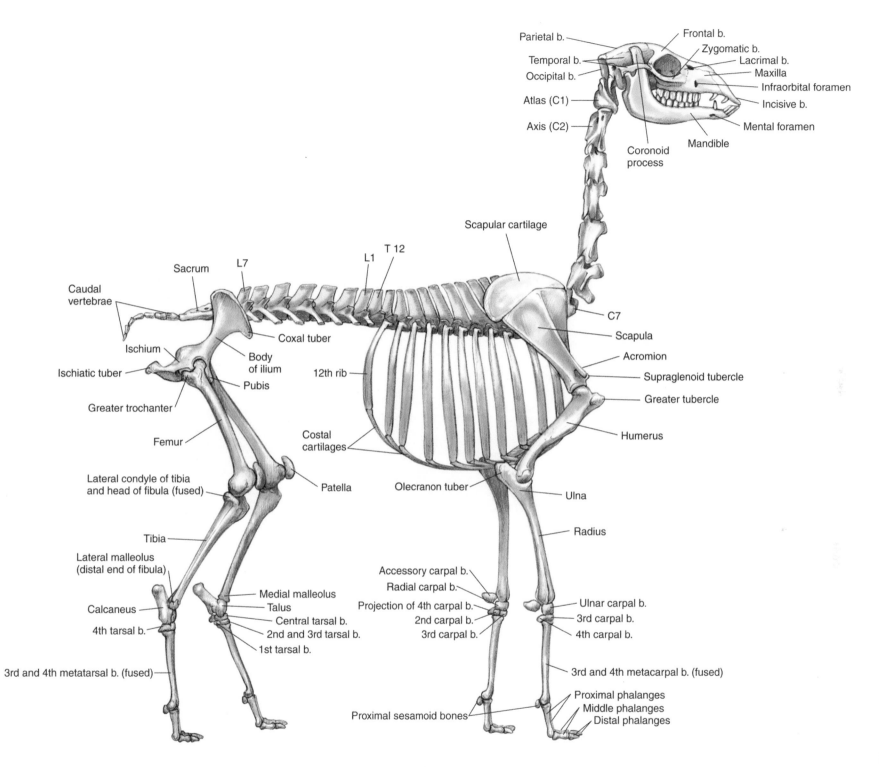

PLATE 5.4 Skeleton of the llama. Right lateral view. C = cervical vertebra, T = thoracic vertebra, L = lumbar vetebra, b = bone

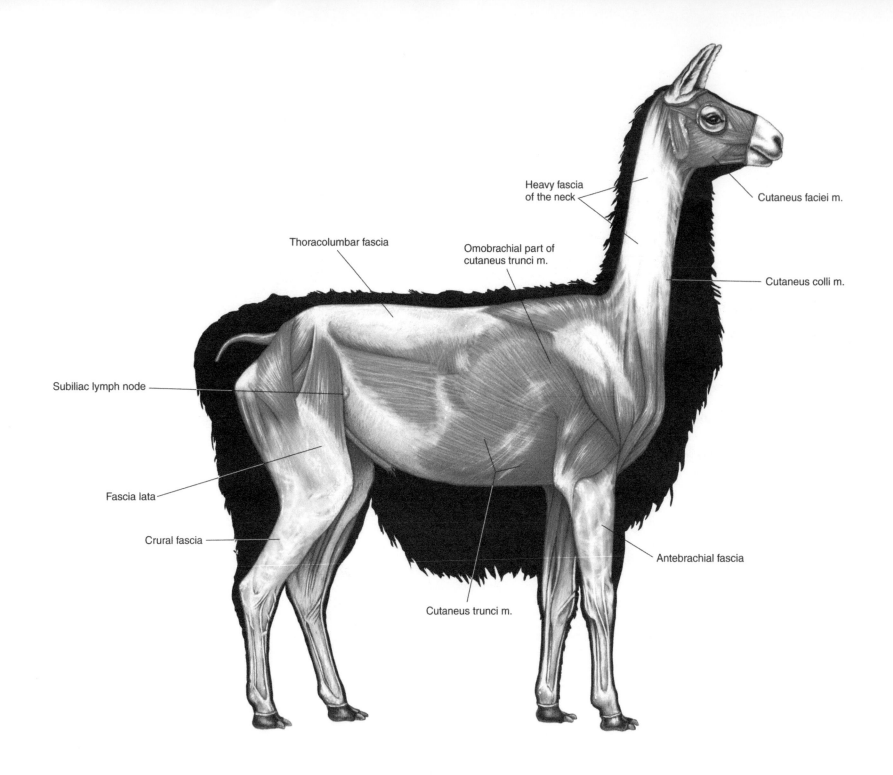

Heavy fascia
of the neck

Cutaneus faciei m.

Thoracolumbar fascia

Omobrachial part of
cutaneus trunci m.

Cutaneus colli m.

Subiliac lymph node

Fascia lata

Crural fascia

Antebrachial fascia

Cutaneus trunci m.

94

PLATE 5.5 Cutaneous muscles and major fasciae of the male llama.
Right lateral view. m = muscle

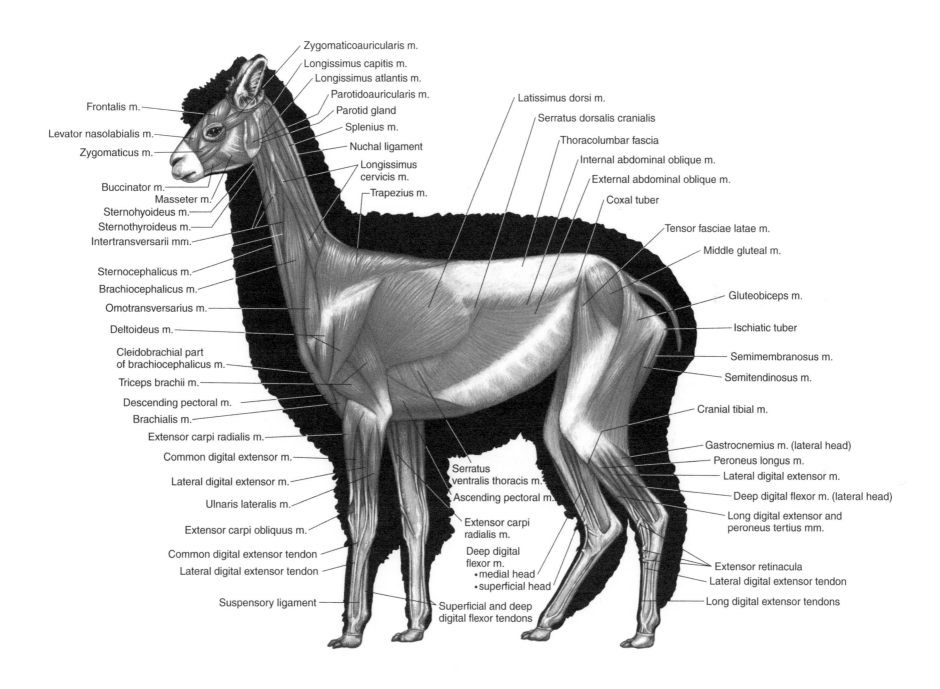

Zygomaticoauricularis m.

Longissimus capitis m.

Longissimus atlantis m.

Parotidoauricularis m.

Frontalis m.

Parotid gland

Levator nasolabialis m.

Splenius m.

Zygomaticus m.

Nuchal ligament

Longissimus
cervicis m.

Buccinator m.

Trapezius m.

Masseter m.

Sternohyoideus m.

Sternothyroideus m.

Intertransversarii mm.

Sternocephalicus m.

Brachiocephalicus m.

Omotransversarius m.

Deltoideus m.

Cleidobrachial part
of brachiocephalicus m.

Triceps brachii m.

Descending pectoral m.

Brachialis m.

Extensor carpi radialis m.

Common digital extensor m.

Lateral digital extensor m.

Ulnaris lateralis m.

Extensor carpi obliquus m.

Common digital extensor tendon

Lateral digital extensor tendon

Suspensory ligament

Latissimus dorsi m.

Serratus dorsalis cranialis

Thoracolumbar fascia

Internal abdominal oblique m.

External abdominal oblique m.

Coxal tuber

Tensor fasciae latae m.

Middle gluteal m.

Gluteobiceps m.

Ischiatic tuber

Semimembranosus m.

Semitendinosus m.

Cranial tibial m.

Gastrocnemius m. (lateral head)

Peroneus longus m.

Lateral digital extensor m.

Deep digital flexor m. (lateral head)

Long digital extensor and
peroneus tertius mm.

Extensor retinacula

Lateral digital extensor tendon

Long digital extensor tendons

Serratus
ventralis thoracis m.

Ascending pectoral m.

Extensor carpi
radialis m.

Deep digital
flexor m.
 •medial head
 •superficial head

Superficial and deep
digital flexor tendons

95

PLATE 5.6 Superficial muscles of the female alpaca. Left lateral view. m = muscle

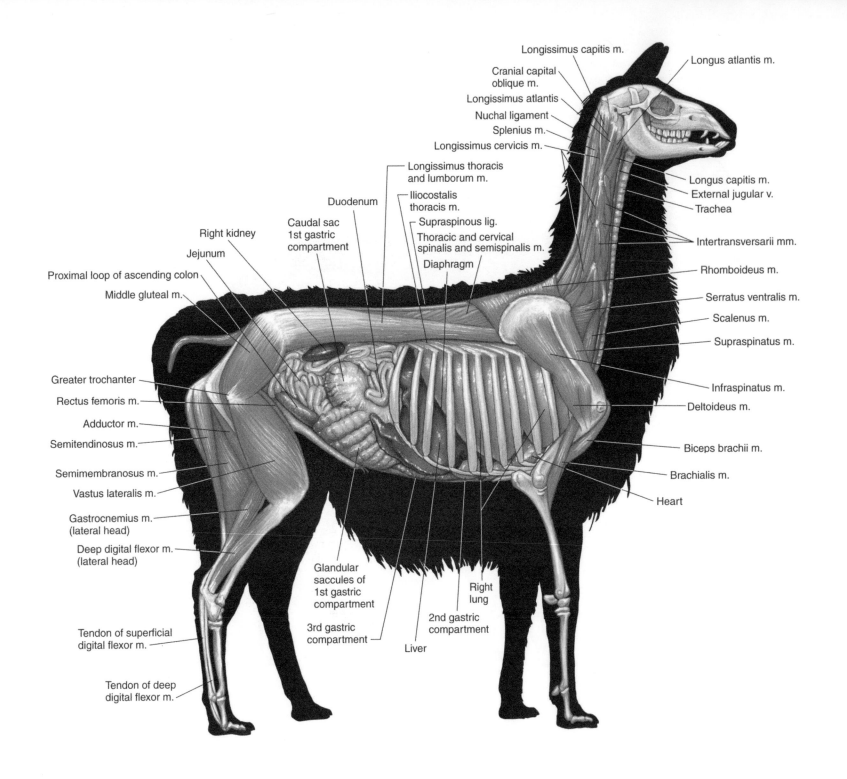

Longissimus capitis m.

Longus atlantis m.

Cranial capital
oblique m.

Longissimus atlantis

Nuchal ligament

Splenius m.

Longissimus cervicis m.

Longissimus thoracis
and lumborum m.

Duodenum

Iliocostalis
thoracis m.

Caudal sac
1st gastric
compartment

Supraspinous lig.

Thoracic and cervical
spinalis and semispinalis m.

Right kidney

Diaphragm

Longus capitis m.

External jugular v.

Trachea

Intertransversarii mm.

Jejunum

Rhomboideus m.

Proximal loop of ascending colon

Serratus ventralis m.

Middle gluteal m.

Scalenus m.

Supraspinatus m.

Greater trochanter

Infraspinatus m.

Rectus femoris m.

Deltoideus m.

Adductor m.

Semitendinosus m.

Biceps brachii m.

Semimembranosus m.

Brachialis m.

Vastus lateralis m.

Heart

Gastrocnemius m.
(lateral head)

Deep digital flexor m.
(lateral head)

Glandular
saccules of
1st gastric
compartment

Right
lung

3rd gastric
compartment

2nd gastric
compartment

Tendon of superficial
digital flexor m.

Liver

Tendon of deep
digital flexor m.

96

PLATE 5.7   Deep muscles and *in situ* viscera of the male llama. Omentum is removed.
Right lateral view. m = muscle, v = vein, lig = ligament

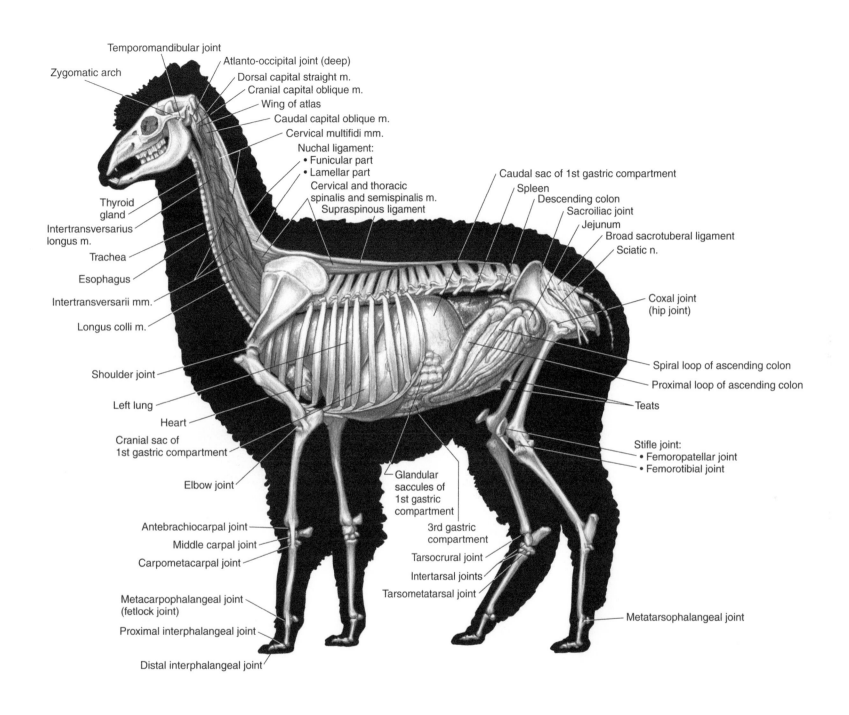

Temporomandibular joint

Zygomatic arch

Atlanto-occipital joint (deep)

Dorsal capital straight m.

Cranial capital oblique m.

Wing of atlas

Caudal capital oblique m.

Cervical multifidi mm.

Nuchal ligament:
• Funicular part
• Lamellar part

Cervical and thoracic
spinalis and semispinalis m.

Supraspinous ligament

Caudal sac of 1st gastric compartment

Spleen

Descending colon

Sacroiliac joint

Jejunum

Broad sacrotuberal ligament

Sciatic n.

Thyroid gland

Intertransversarius longus m.

Trachea

Esophagus

Intertransversarii mm.

Longus colli m.

Coxal joint (hip joint)

Shoulder joint

Left lung

Heart

Cranial sac of 1st gastric compartment

Elbow joint

Spiral loop of ascending colon

Proximal loop of ascending colon

Teats

Stifle joint:
• Femoropatellar joint
• Femorotibial joint

Glandular saccules of 1st gastric compartment

3rd gastric compartment

Antebrachiocarpal joint

Middle carpal joint

Carpometacarpal joint

Tarsocrural joint

Intertarsal joints

Tarsometatarsal joint

Metacarpophalangeal joint (fetlock joint)

Proximal interphalangeal joint

Metatarsophalangeal joint

Distal interphalangeal joint

PLATE 5.8   Deep cervical muscles, *in situ* viscera, and major joints of the female alpaca.
The omentum is removed. Left lateral view. m = muscle

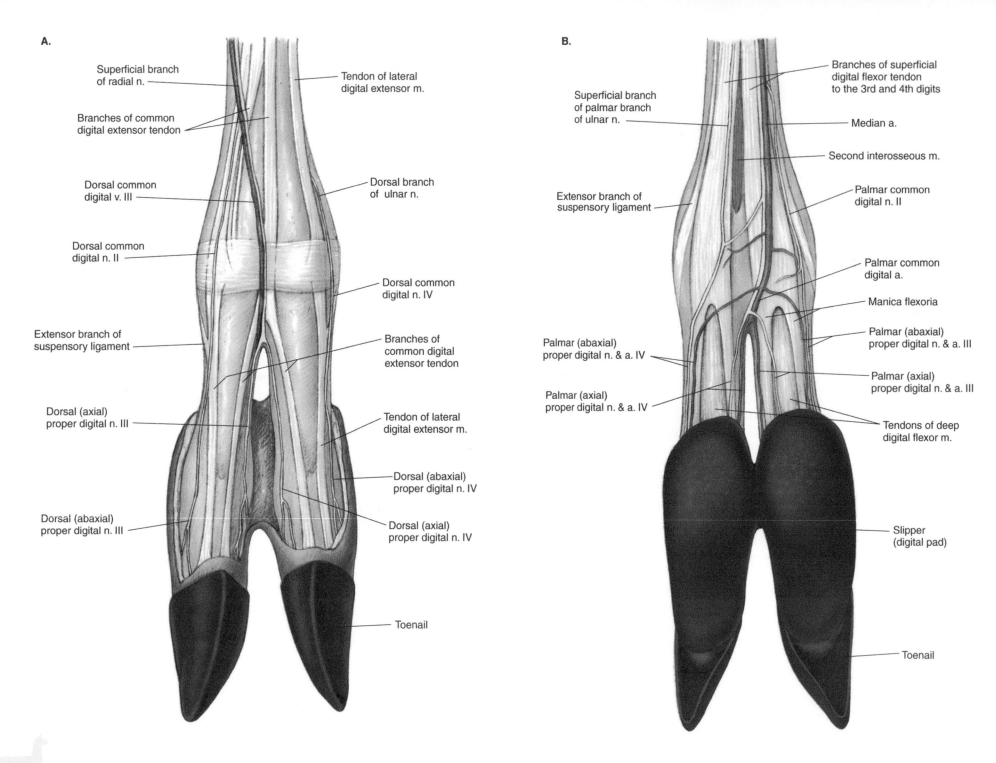

A.

Superficial branch of radial n.

Branches of common digital extensor tendon

Dorsal common digital v. III

Dorsal common digital n. II

Extensor branch of suspensory ligament

Dorsal (axial) proper digital n. III

Dorsal (abaxial) proper digital n. III

Tendon of lateral digital extensor m.

Dorsal branch of ulnar n.

Dorsal common digital n. IV

Branches of common digital extensor tendon

Tendon of lateral digital extensor m.

Dorsal (abaxial) proper digital n. IV

Dorsal (axial) proper digital n. IV

Toenail

B.

Superficial branch of palmar branch of ulnar n.

Extensor branch of suspensory ligament

Palmar (abaxial) proper digital n. & a. IV

Palmar (axial) proper digital n. & a. IV

Branches of superficial digital flexor tendon to the 3rd and 4th digits

Median a.

Second interosseous m.

Palmar common digital n. II

Palmar common digital a.

Manica flexoria

Palmar (abaxial) proper digital n. & a. III

Palmar (axial) proper digital n. & a. III

Tendons of deep digital flexor m.

Slipper (digital pad)

Toenail

PLATE 5.9 Major structures of the lamoid left distal metacarpus and digits. **A.** Dorsal view.
B. Palmar view. n = nerve, v = vein, m = muscle, a = artery

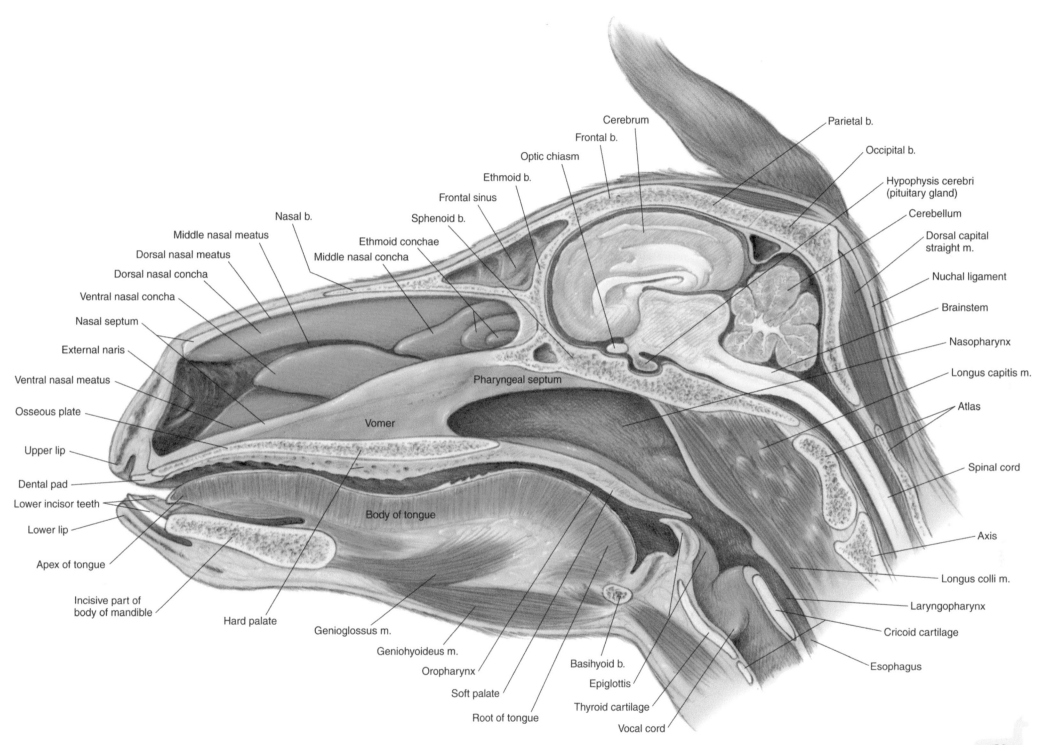

Cerebrum

Frontal b.

Optic chiasm

Ethmoid b.

Frontal sinus

Sphenoid b.

Ethmoid conchae

Middle nasal concha

Nasal b.

Middle nasal meatus

Dorsal nasal meatus

Dorsal nasal concha

Ventral nasal concha

Nasal septum

External naris

Ventral nasal meatus

Osseous plate

Upper lip

Dental pad

Lower incisor teeth

Lower lip

Apex of tongue

Incisive part of
body of mandible

Hard palate

Genioglossus m.

Geniohyoideus m.

Oropharynx

Soft palate

Root of tongue

Basihyoid b.

Epiglottis

Thyroid cartilage

Vocal cord

Vomer

Body of tongue

Pharyngeal septum

Parietal b.

Occipital b.

Hypophysis cerebri
(pituitary gland)

Cerebellum

Dorsal capital
straight m.

Nuchal ligament

Brainstem

Nasopharynx

Longus capitis m.

Atlas

Spinal cord

Axis

Longus colli m.

Laryngopharynx

Cricoid cartilage

Esophagus

PLATE 5.10   Median section of the llama's head. Most of the
nasal septum is removed. b = bone, m = muscle

99

A.

Outline of
skull bones

Nostril

B.

Outline of
skull bones

Nostril

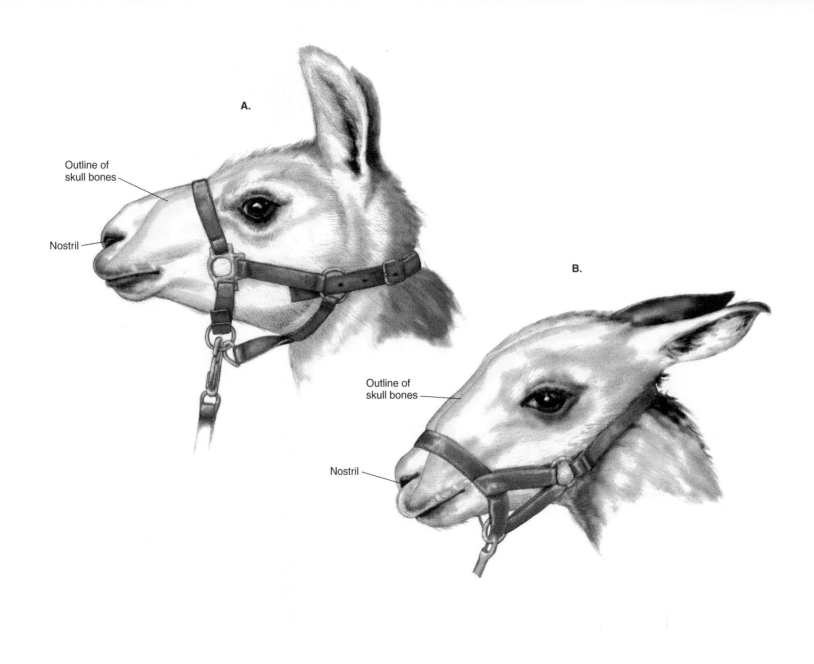

100

PLATE 5.11   A. Proper placement of a halter on a llama's head. B. Improper placement
of a halter. Pressure on the nostrils interferes with breathing.

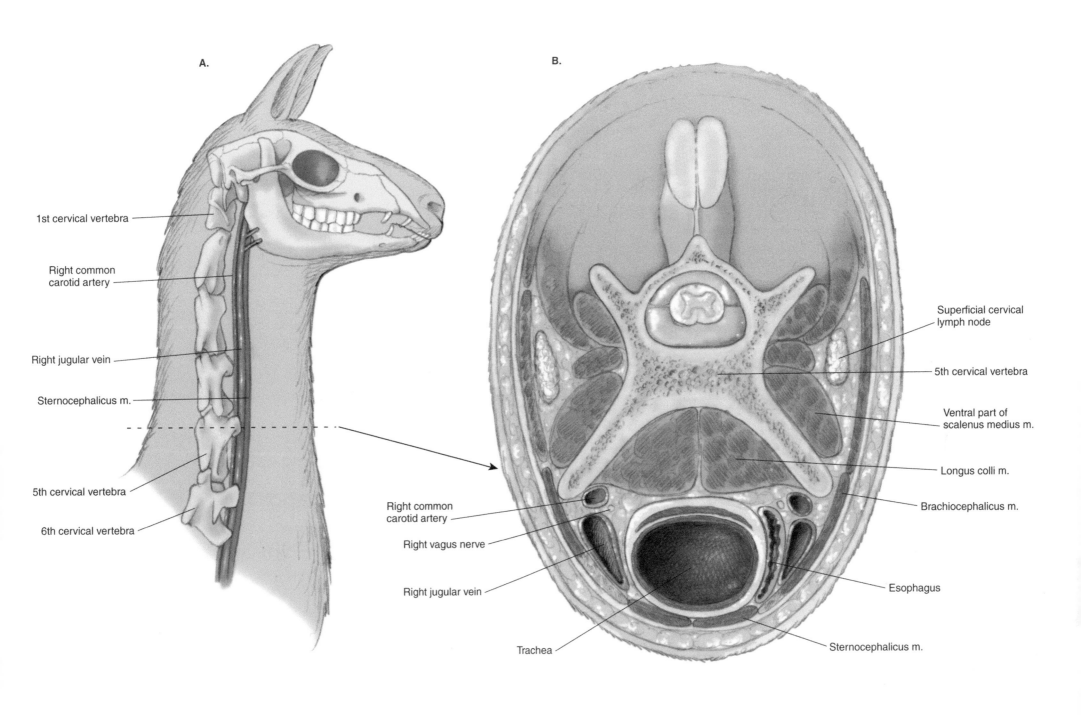

A.

B.

1st cervical vertebra

Right common
carotid artery

Right jugular vein

Sternocephalicus m.

5th cervical vertebra

6th cervical vertebra

Superficial cervical
lymph node

5th cervical vertebra

Ventral part of
scalenus medius m.

Longus colli m.

Brachiocephalicus m.

Esophagus

Sternocephalicus m.

Right common
carotid artery

Right vagus nerve

Right jugular vein

Trachea

PLATE 5.12 Relations of the llama's common carotid artery and jugular vein. **A.** Right
lateral view of the head and neck. **B.** Cross-section through the neck at the
level of the 5th cervical vertebra. m = muscle

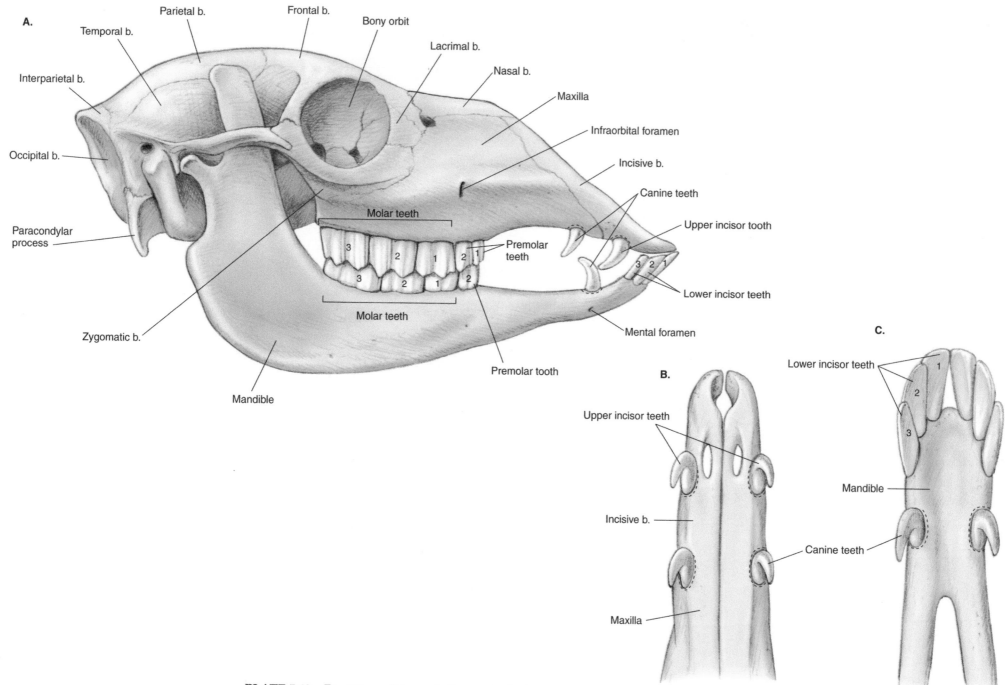

A.

Parietal b.

Frontal b.

Temporal b.

Bony orbit

Lacrimal b.

Interparietal b.

Nasal b.

Maxilla

Occipital b.

Infraorbital foramen

Incisive b.

Canine teeth

Paracondylar
process

Molar teeth

Upper incisor tooth

3   2   1   2   1

Premolar
teeth

3   2   1   2

3 2 1

Lower incisor teeth

Molar teeth

Zygomatic b.

Mental foramen

Premolar tooth

Mandible

C.

Lower incisor teeth

B.

1

Upper incisor teeth

2

3

Incisive b.

Mandible

Canine teeth

Canine teeth

Maxilla

PLATE 5.13   Dentition of the male llama. **A.** Right lateral view of the skull and crowns of
permanent teeth *in situ*. **B.** Ventral view of the crowns of the upper incisor and canine
teeth. **C.** Dorsal view of the crowns of the lower incisor and canine teeth. *Dashed
lines* indicate the plane of sectioning (2–3 mm above the gum [gingival] line)
for cutting off the crowns of deciduous or erupting permanent
canine and upper incisor teeth. b = bone

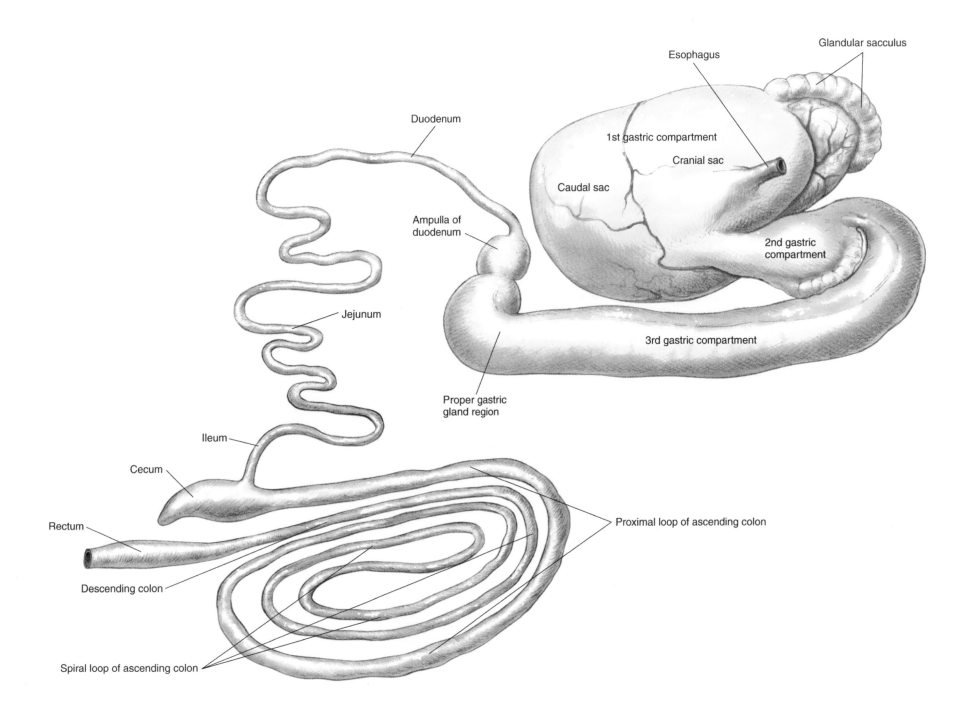

Esophagus

Glandular sacculus

Duodenum

1st gastric compartment

Cranial sac

Caudal sac

2nd gastric compartment

Ampulla of duodenum

Jejunum

3rd gastric compartment

Proper gastric gland region

Ileum

Cecum

Proximal loop of ascending colon

Rectum

Descending colon

Spiral loop of ascending colon

103

PLATE 5.14   Isolated stomach and intestines of the male llama. Jejunum is shortened.

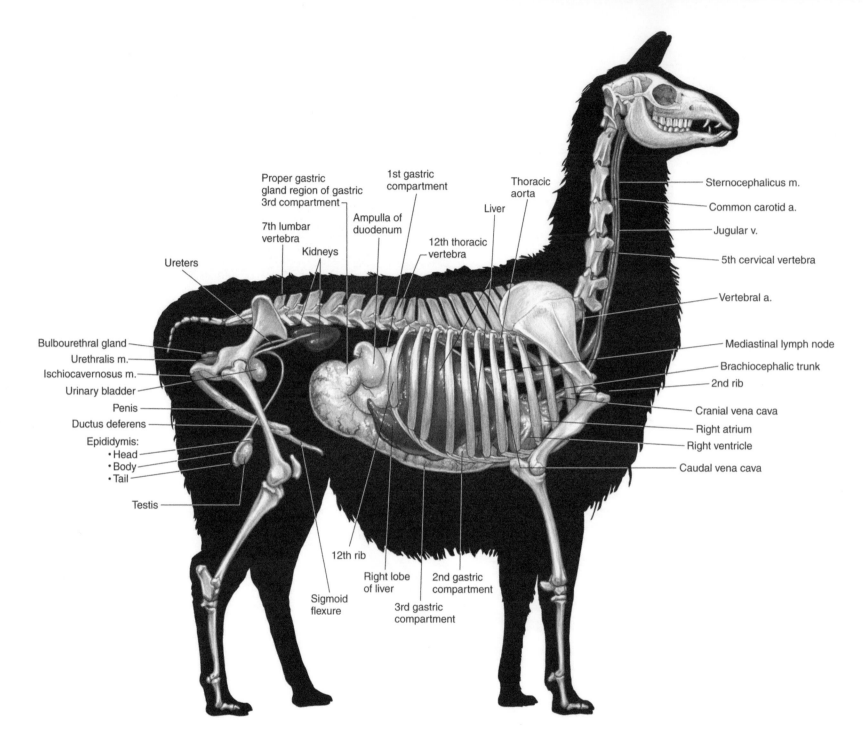

Proper gastric
gland region of gastric
3rd compartment

1st gastric
compartment

Thoracic
aorta

Sternocephalicus m.

Common carotid a.

Ampulla of
duodenum

Liver

7th lumbar
vertebra

Jugular v.

12th thoracic
vertebra

Kidneys

5th cervical vertebra

Ureters

Vertebral a.

Bulbourethral gland

Mediastinal lymph node

Urethralis m.

Brachiocephalic trunk

Ischiocavernosus m.

2nd rib

Urinary bladder

Cranial vena cava

Penis

Right atrium

Ductus deferens

Right ventricle

Epididymis:
• Head

Caudal vena cava

• Body
• Tail

Testis

12th rib

Right lobe
of liver

2nd gastric
compartment

Sigmoid
flexure

3rd gastric
compartment

PLATE 5.15   Reproductive and urinary organs, stomach, liver, heart, and adjacent major
vessels related to the skeleton of the male llama. Lungs and intestines are removed.
Right lateral view. v = vein, a = artery, m = muscle

104

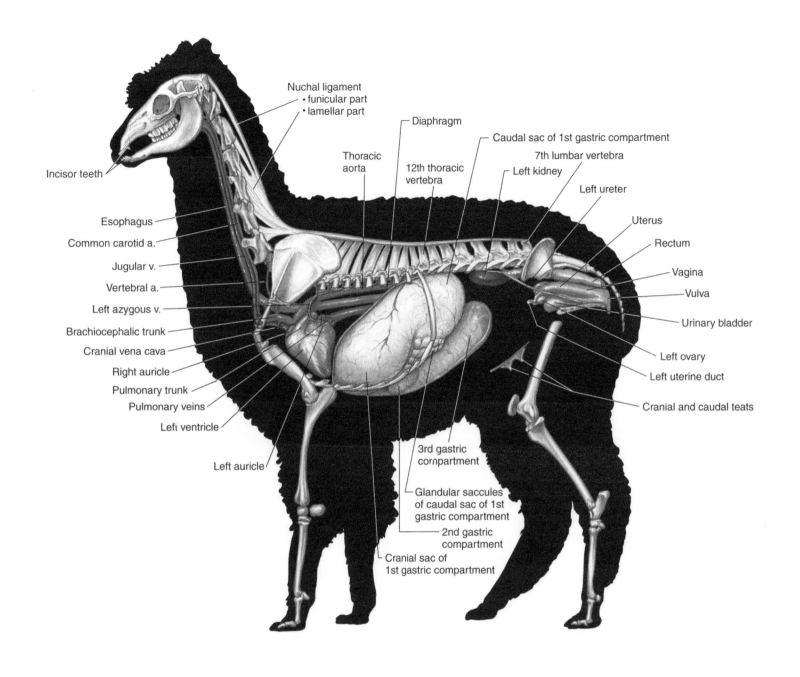

Nuchal ligament
• funicular part
• lamellar part

Diaphragm

Caudal sac of 1st gastric compartment

7th lumbar vertebra

Thoracic
aorta

12th thoracic
vertebra

Left kidney

Left ureter

Incisor teeth

Uterus

Esophagus

Rectum

Common carotid a.

Vagina

Jugular v.

Vulva

Vertebral a.

Left azygous v.

Urinary bladder

Brachiocephalic trunk

Cranial vena cava

Right auricle

Left ovary

Pulmonary trunk

Left uterine duct

Pulmonary veins

Left ventricle

Cranial and caudal teats

Left auricle

3rd gastric
compartment

Glandular saccules
of caudal sac of 1st
gastric compartment

2nd gastric
compartment

Cranial sac of
1st gastric compartment

PLATE 5.16   Reproductive and urinary organs, stomach, heart, and adjacent major
vessels of the female alpaca. Lungs and intestines are removed. Left
lateral view. a = artery, v = vein

105

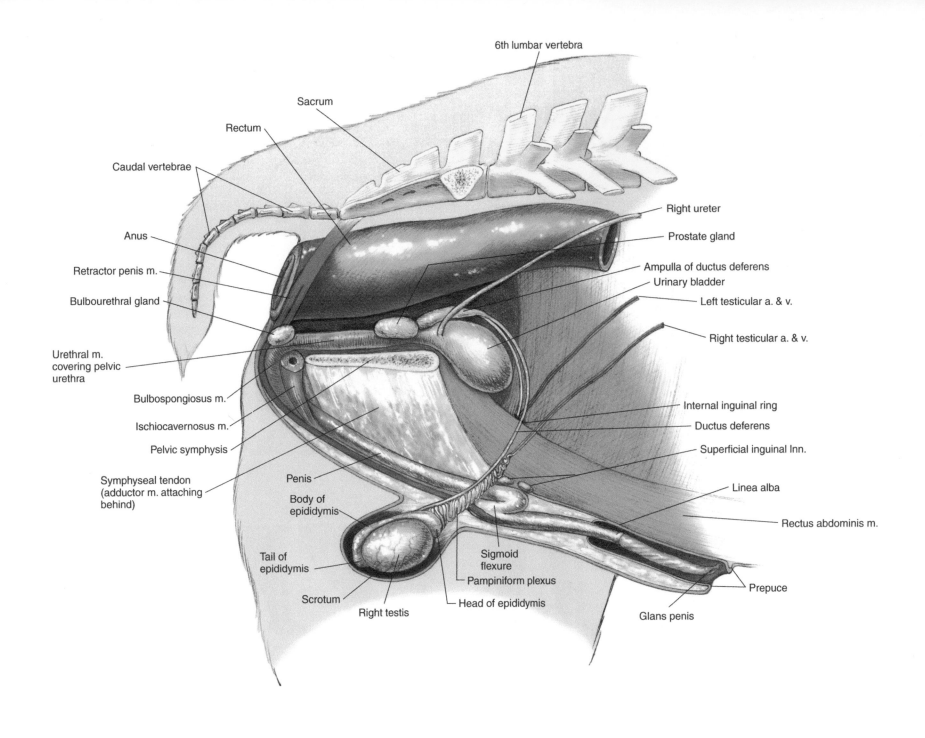

6th lumbar vertebra

Sacrum

Rectum

Caudal vertebrae

Anus

Retractor penis m.

Bulbourethral gland

Urethral m.
covering pelvic
urethra

Bulbospongiosus m.

Ischiocavernosus m.

Pelvic symphysis

Symphyseal tendon
(adductor m. attaching
behind)

Penis

Body of
epididymis

Tail of
epididymis

Scrotum

Right testis

Sigmoid
flexure

Pampiniform plexus

Head of epididymis

Right ureter

Prostate gland

Ampulla of ductus deferens

Urinary bladder

Left testicular a. & v.

Right testicular a. & v.

Internal inguinal ring

Ductus deferens

Superficial inguinal lnn.

Linea alba

Rectus abdominis m.

Prepuce

Glans penis

106

PLATE 5.17 Relations of the reproductive organs of the male llama. Right lateral view.
m = muscle, lnn = lymph nodes, v = vein, a = artery

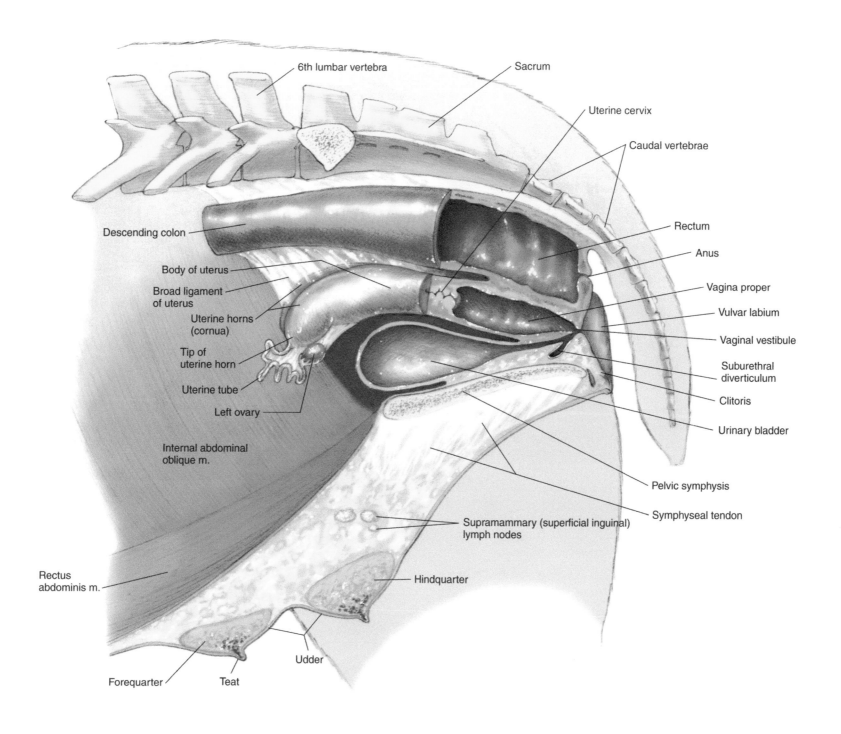

6th lumbar vertebra

Sacrum

Uterine cervix

Caudal vertebrae

Descending colon

Rectum

Anus

Body of uterus

Broad ligament
of uterus

Uterine horns
(cornua)

Tip of
uterine horn

Uterine tube

Left ovary

Internal abdominal
oblique m.

Vagina proper

Vulvar labium

Vaginal vestibule

Suburethral
diverticulum

Clitoris

Urinary bladder

Pelvic symphysis

Symphyseal tendon

Supramammary (superficial inguinal)
lymph nodes

Rectus
abdominis m.

Hindquarter

Forequarter

Teat

Udder

PLATE 5.18 Relations of the reproductive organs of the female alpaca.
Partial median section. Left lateral view. m = muscle

SECTION 6 THE SWINE *(Sus scrofa domesticus)*

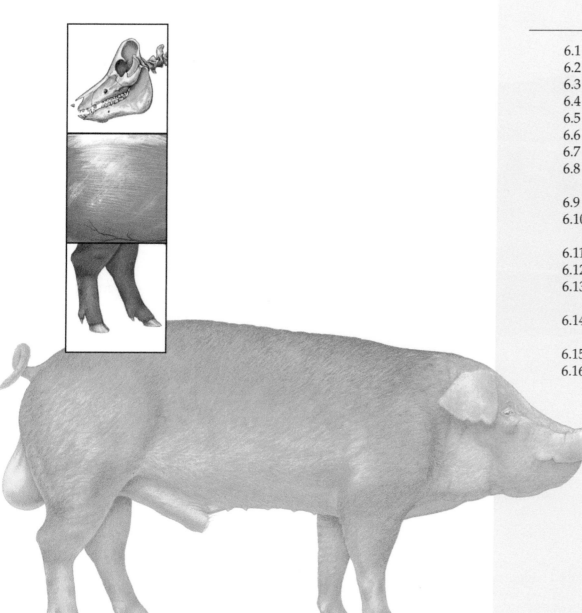

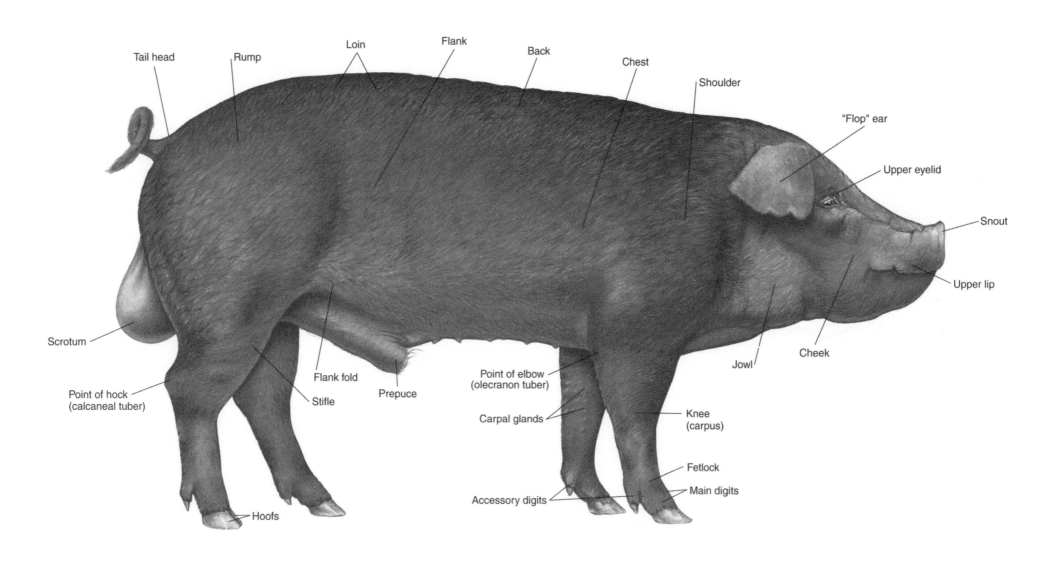

PLATE 6.1 Right lateral view of a boar.

Tail head

Rump

Loin

Flank

Back

Chest

Shoulder

"Flop" ear

Upper eyelid

Snout

Upper lip

Cheek

Jowl

Knee (carpus)

Fetlock

Main digits

Accessory digits

Point of elbow (olecranon tuber)

Carpal glands

Prepuce

Stifle

Flank fold

Point of hock (calcaneal tuber)

Scrotum

Hoofs

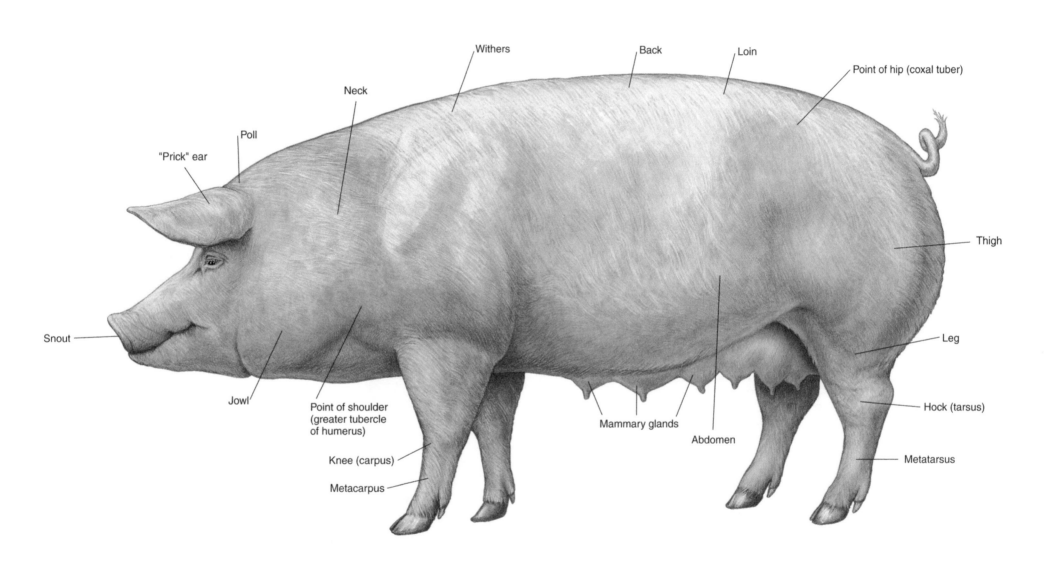

Withers

Back

Loin

Point of hip (coxal tuber)

Neck

Poll

"Prick" ear

Thigh

Snout

Leg

Jowl

Point of shoulder
(greater tubercle
of humerus)

Mammary glands

Abdomen

Hock (tarsus)

Knee (carpus)

Metatarsus

Metacarpus

PLATE 6.2   Left lateral view of a sow.

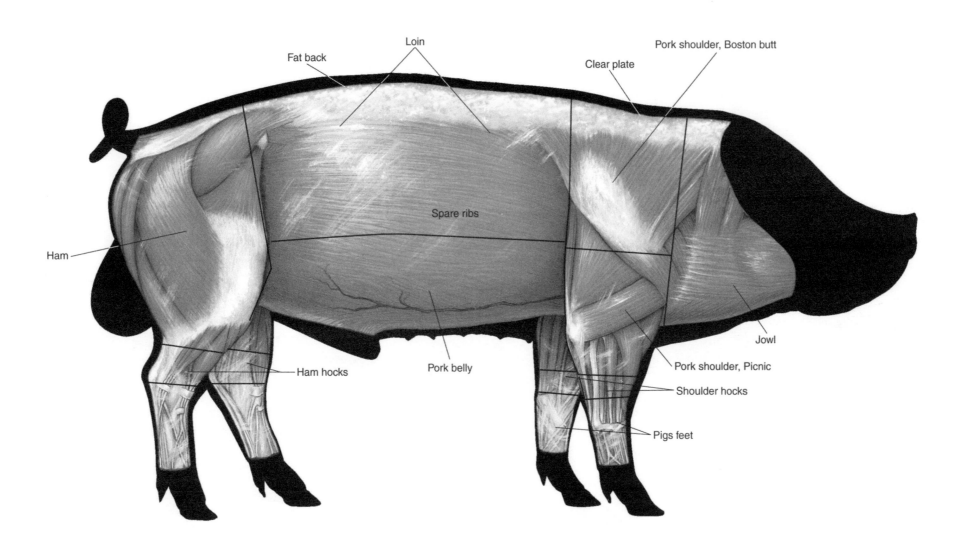

PLATE 6.3 Carcass cuts of the hog.

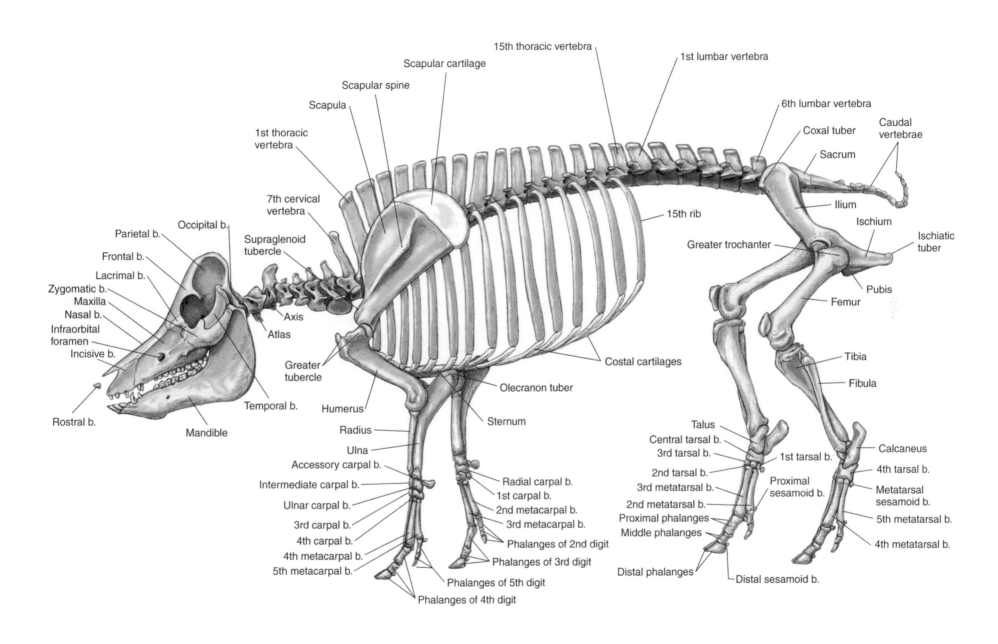

15th thoracic vertebra

1st lumbar vertebra

Scapular cartilage

6th lumbar vertebra

Scapular spine

Caudal vertebrae

Scapula

Coxal tuber

1st thoracic vertebra

Sacrum

7th cervical vertebra

Ilium

Parietal b.

Occipital b.

Supraglenoid tubercle

15th rib

Frontal b.

Ischium

Lacrimal b.

Ischiatic tuber

Zygomatic b.

Greater trochanter

Maxilla

Axis

Pubis

Nasal b.

Atlas

Femur

Infraorbital foramen

Incisive b.

Greater tubercle

Costal cartilages

Tibia

Rostral b.

Olecranon tuber

Fibula

Temporal b.

Humerus

Mandible

Radius

Sternum

Ulna

Talus

Accessory carpal b.

Radial carpal b.

Central tarsal b.

Calcaneus

Intermediate carpal b.

1st carpal b.

3rd tarsal b.

1st tarsal b.

4th tarsal b.

Ulnar carpal b.

2nd metacarpal b.

2nd tarsal b.

Proximal sesamoid b.

Metatarsal sesamoid b.

3rd carpal b.

3rd metacarpal b.

3rd metatarsal b.

4th carpal b.

Phalanges of 2nd digit

2nd metatarsal b.

5th metatarsal b.

4th metacarpal b.

Phalanges of 3rd digit

Proximal phalanges

5th metacarpal b.

Middle phalanges

4th metatarsal b.

Phalanges of 5th digit

Distal phalanges

Distal sesamoid b.

Phalanges of 4th digit

PLATE 6.4   Skeleton of the swine. b = bone

113

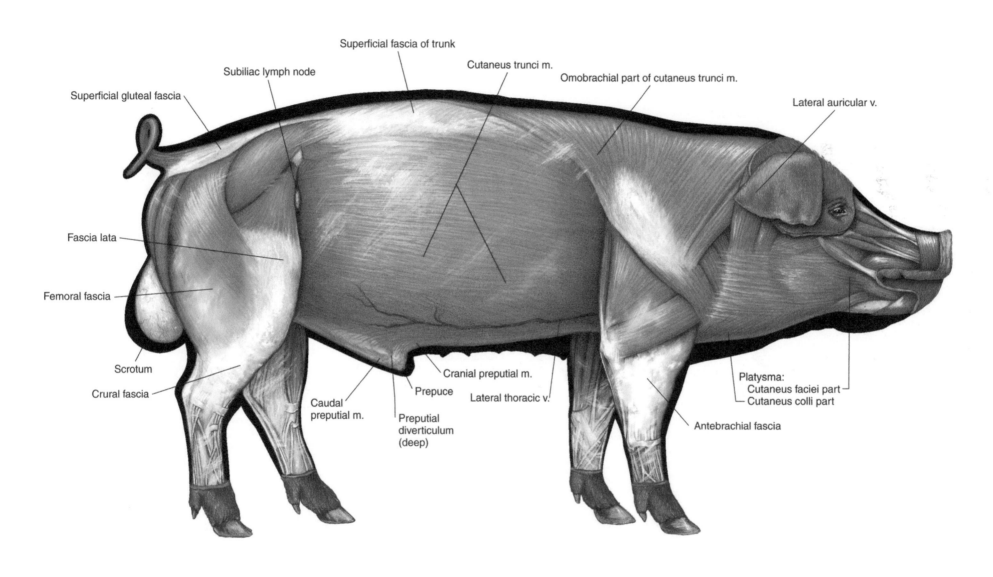

Superficial fascia of trunk

Subiliac lymph node

Cutaneus trunci m.

Omobrachial part of cutaneus trunci m.

Lateral auricular v.

Superficial gluteal fascia

Fascia lata

Femoral fascia

Scrotum

Crural fascia

Caudal preputial m.

Preputial diverticulum (deep)

Prepuce

Cranial preputial m.

Lateral thoracic v.

Platysma:
Cutaneus faciei part
Cutaneus colli part

Antebrachial fascia

PLATE 6.5   Cutaneous and superficial muscles of the boar. Panniculus adiposus (fat layer) removed. Right lateral view. v = vein, m = muscle

114

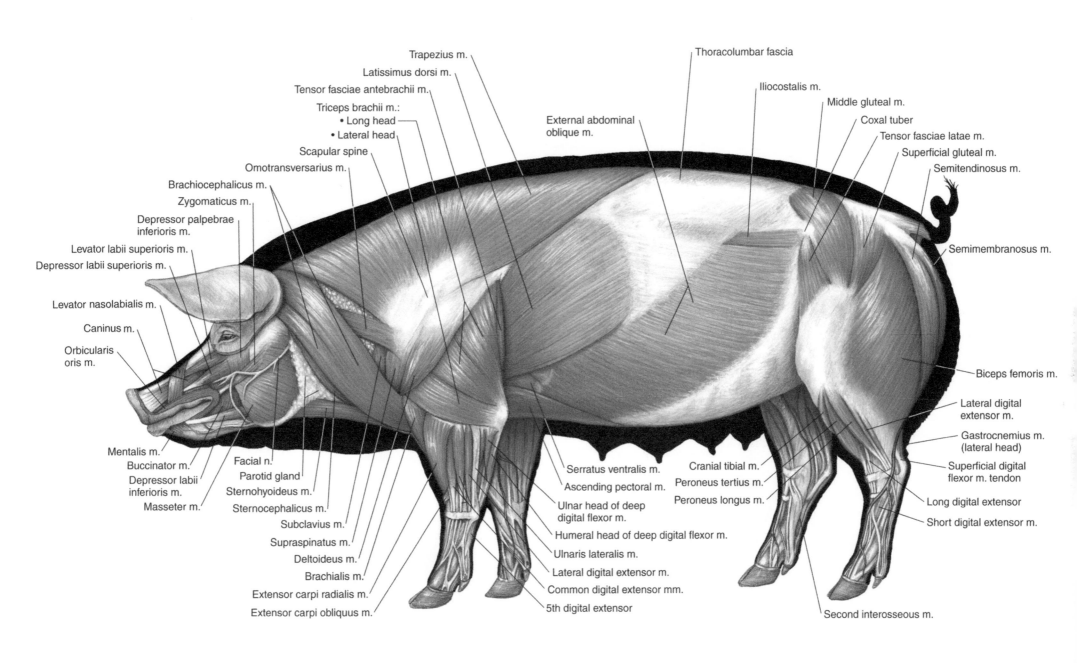

Trapezius m.

Latissimus dorsi m.

Tensor fasciae antebrachii m.

Triceps brachii m.:
• Long head
• Lateral head

Scapular spine

Omotransversarius m.

Brachiocephalicus m.

Zygomaticus m.

Depressor palpebrae inferioris m.

Levator labii superioris m.

Depressor labii superioris m.

Levator nasolabialis m.

Caninus m.

Orbicularis oris m.

Mentalis m.

Buccinator m.

Depressor labii inferioris m.

Masseter m.

Facial n.

Parotid gland

Sternohyoideus m.

Sternocephalicus m.

Subclavius m.

Supraspinatus m.

Deltoideus m.

Brachialis m.

Extensor carpi radialis m.

Extensor carpi obliquus m.

External abdominal oblique m.

Serratus ventralis m.

Ascending pectoral m.

Ulnar head of deep digital flexor m.

Humeral head of deep digital flexor m.

Ulnaris lateralis m.

Lateral digital extensor m.

Common digital extensor mm.

5th digital extensor

Thoracolumbar fascia

Iliocostalis m.

Middle gluteal m.

Coxal tuber

Tensor fasciae latae m.

Superficial gluteal m.

Semitendinosus m.

Semimembranosus m.

Biceps femoris m.

Lateral digital extensor m.

Gastrocnemius m. (lateral head)

Superficial digital flexor m. tendon

Long digital extensor

Short digital extensor m.

Cranial tibial m.

Peroneus tertius m.

Peroneus longus m.

Second interosseous m.

PLATE 6.6   Superficial muscles of the sow. Left lateral view. m = muscle, n = nerve

115

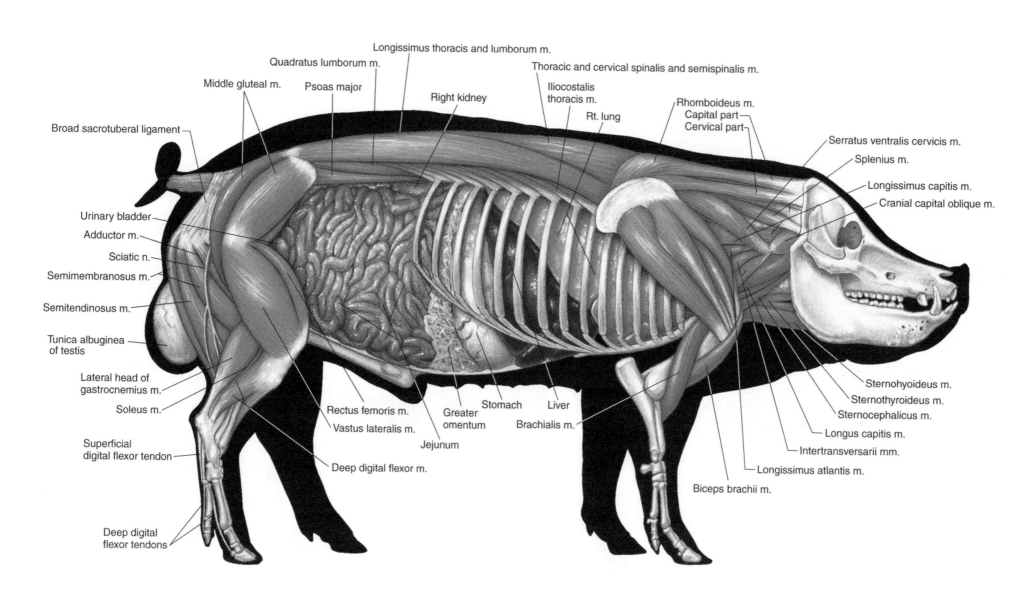

Longissimus thoracis and lumborum m.

Quadratus lumborum m.

Thoracic and cervical spinalis and semispinalis m.

Middle gluteal m.　　Psoas major

Right kidney

Iliocostalis
thoracis m.

Rhomboideus m.

Rt. lung

Capital part
Cervical part

Broad sacrotuberal ligament

Serratus ventralis cervicis m.

Splenius m.

Longissimus capitis m.

Cranial capital oblique m.

Urinary bladder

Adductor m.

Sciatic n.

Semimembranosus m.

Semitendinosus m.

Tunica albuginea
of testis

Lateral head of
gastrocnemius m.

Soleus m.

Superficial
digital flexor tendon

Rectus femoris m.

Vastus lateralis m.

Deep digital flexor m.

Jejunum

Greater
omentum

Stomach　　Liver

Brachialis m.

Sternohyoideus m.

Sternothyroideus m.

Sternocephalicus m.

Longus capitis m.

Intertransversarii mm.

Longissimus atlantis m.

Biceps brachii m.

Deep digital
flexor tendons

PLATE 6.7　Deep muscles and *in situ* viscera of the boar.
Right lateral view. m = muscle, n = nerve

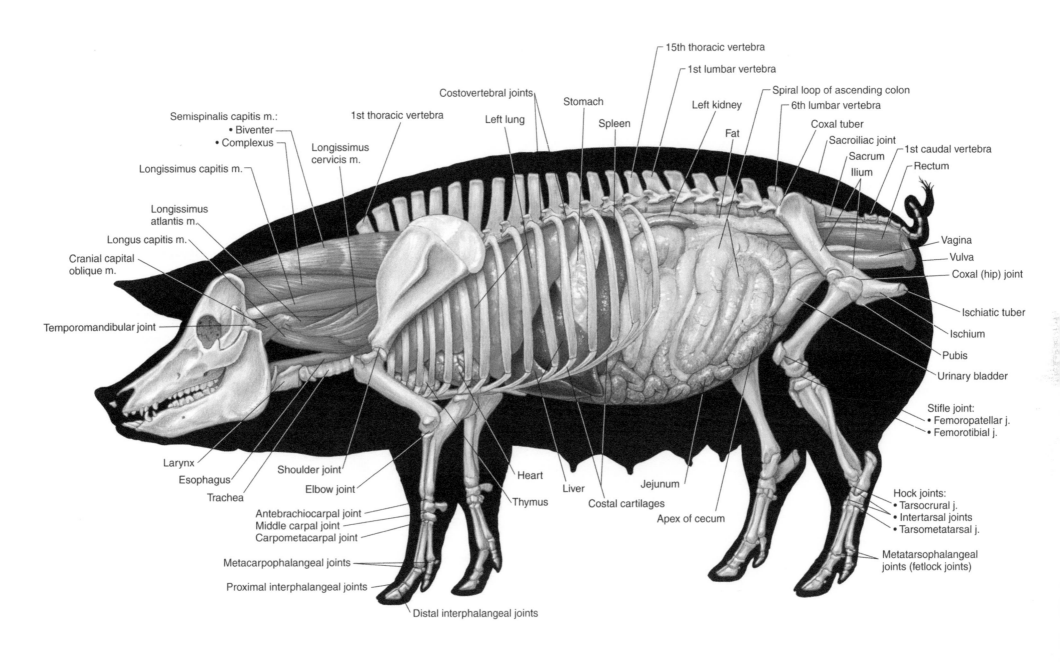

Semispinalis capitis m.:
• Biventer
• Complexus

Longissimus capitis m.

Longissimus atlantis m.

Longus capitis m.

Cranial capital oblique m.

Temporomandibular joint

Longissimus cervicis m.

1st thoracic vertebra

Costovertebral joints

Left lung

Stomach

Spleen

15th thoracic vertebra

1st lumbar vertebra

Spiral loop of ascending colon

Left kidney

6th lumbar vertebra

Fat

Coxal tuber

Sacroiliac joint

Sacrum

Ilium

1st caudal vertebra

Rectum

Vagina

Vulva

Coxal (hip) joint

Ischiatic tuber

Ischium

Pubis

Urinary bladder

Stifle joint:
• Femoropatellar j.
• Femorotibial j.

Hock joints:
• Tarsocrural j.
• Intertarsal joints
• Tarsometatarsal j.

Metatarsophalangeal joints (fetlock joints)

Apex of cecum

Jejunum

Costal cartilages

Liver

Heart

Thymus

Distal interphalangeal joints

Proximal interphalangeal joints

Metacarpophalangeal joints

Carpometacarpal joint

Middle carpal joint

Antebrachiocarpal joint

Elbow joint

Shoulder joint

Trachea

Esophagus

Larynx

PLATE 6.8   Deep cervical muscles, major joints, and *in situ* viscera
of the sow. Left lateral view. m = muscle, j = joint

117

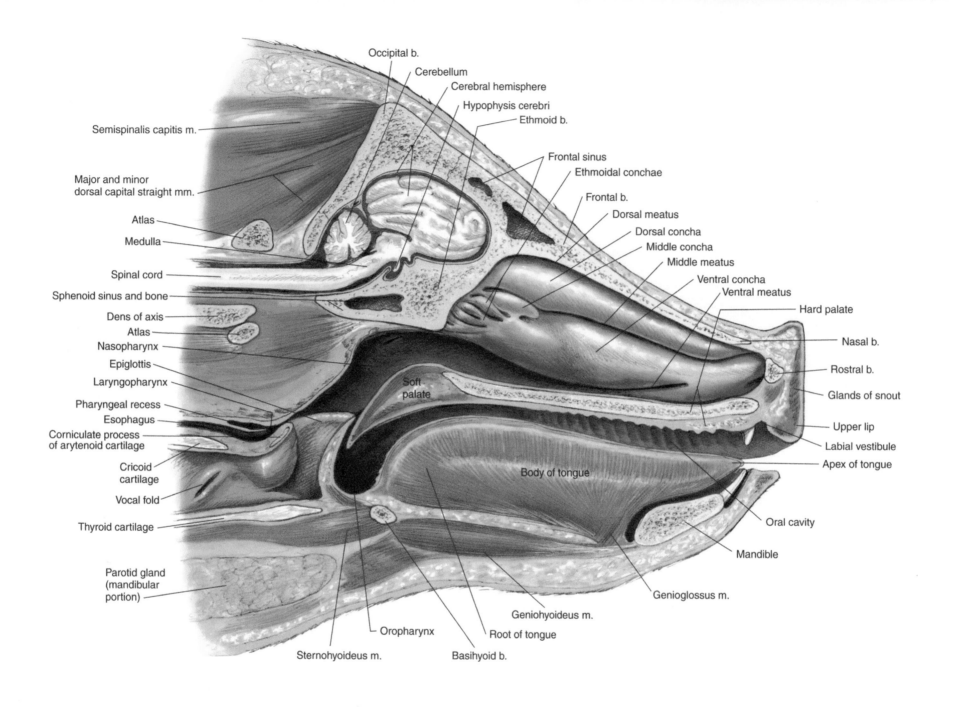

Occipital b.

Cerebellum

Cerebral hemisphere

Hypophysis cerebri

Ethmoid b.

Semispinalis capitis m.

Frontal sinus

Ethmoidal conchae

Major and minor
dorsal capital straight mm.

Frontal b.

Dorsal meatus

Dorsal concha

Atlas

Middle concha

Medulla

Middle meatus

Ventral concha

Spinal cord

Ventral meatus

Sphenoid sinus and bone

Hard palate

Dens of axis

Nasal b.

Atlas

Nasopharynx

Rostral b.

Epiglottis

Glands of snout

Laryngopharynx

Soft
palate

Pharyngeal recess

Upper lip

Esophagus

Labial vestibule

Corniculate process
of arytenoid cartilage

Apex of tongue

Cricoid
cartilage

Body of tongue

Vocal fold

Oral cavity

Thyroid cartilage

Mandible

Parotid gland
(mandibular
portion)

Genioglossus m.

Geniohyoideus m.

Oropharynx

Root of tongue

Sternohyoideus m.

Basihyoid b.

118

PLATE 6.9 Median section of the porcine head. The nasal septum has been removed.
Right lateral view. m = muscle, b = bone

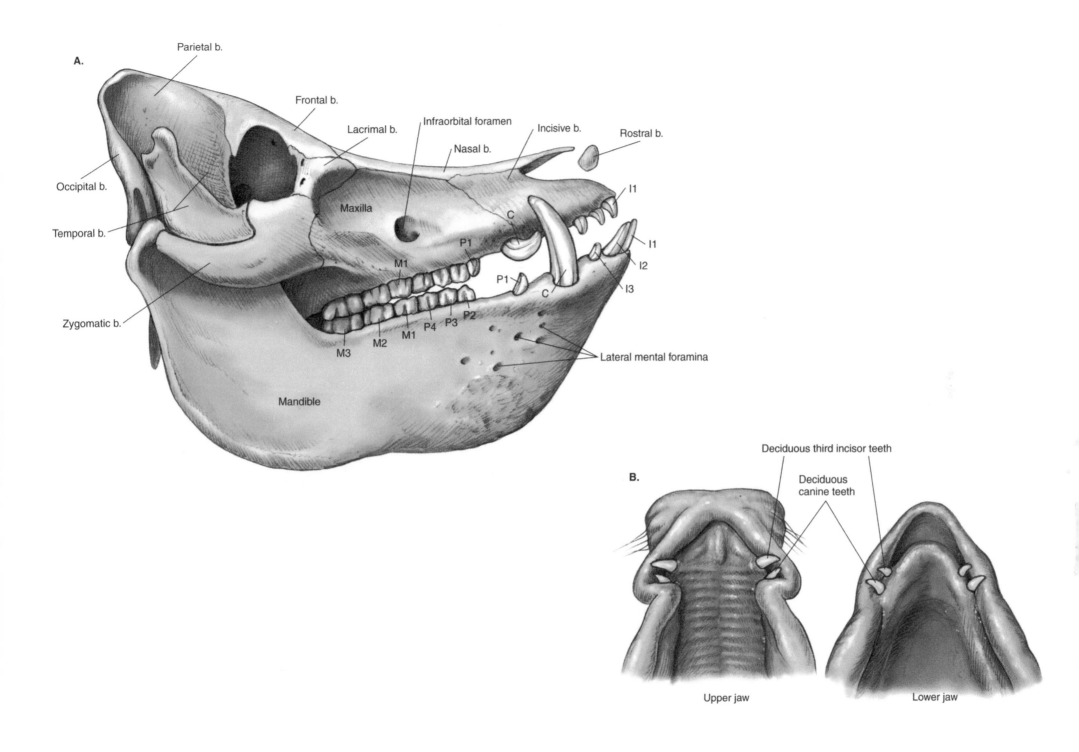

A.

Parietal b.

Frontal b.

Lacrimal b.

Infraorbital foramen

Incisive b.

Nasal b.

Rostral b.

Occipital b.

Temporal b.

Zygomatic b.

Maxilla

I1

C

P1

M1

P1

C

I1

I2

I3

M2

M1

P4 P3 P2

Mandible

M3

Lateral mental foramina

B.

Deciduous third incisor teeth

Deciduous canine teeth

Upper jaw

Lower jaw

PLATE 6.10 **A.** Permanent dentition of the boar. b = bone, I = incisor tooth, C = canine tooth,
P = premolar tooth, M = molar tooth **B.** Cutting the deciduous incisor and canine teeth
of a piglet. They are routinely cut off to prevent damage to sow's teats.

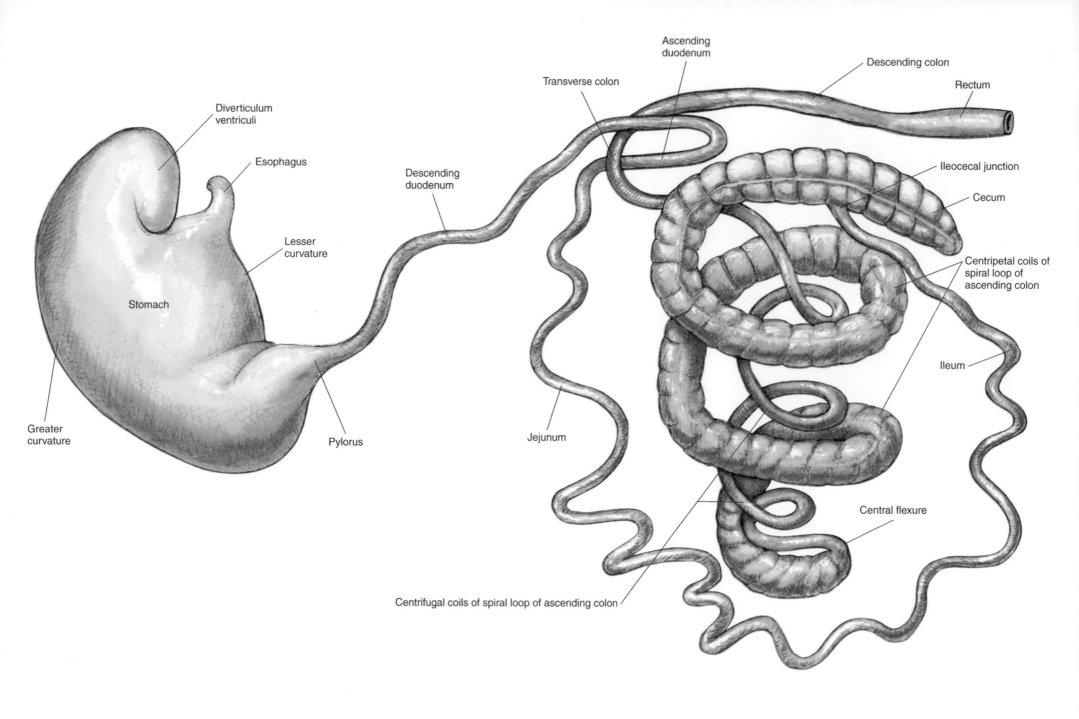

Diverticulum ventriculi

Esophagus

Lesser curvature

Stomach

Greater curvature

Pylorus

Descending duodenum

Transverse colon

Ascending duodenum

Descending colon

Rectum

Ileocecal junction

Cecum

Centripetal coils of spiral loop of ascending colon

Ileum

Jejunum

Centrifugal coils of spiral loop of ascending colon

Central flexure

120

PLATE 6.11   Isolated stomach and intestines of the swine. The jejunum is shortened and uncoiled, and the loops of the ascending colon are pulled apart.

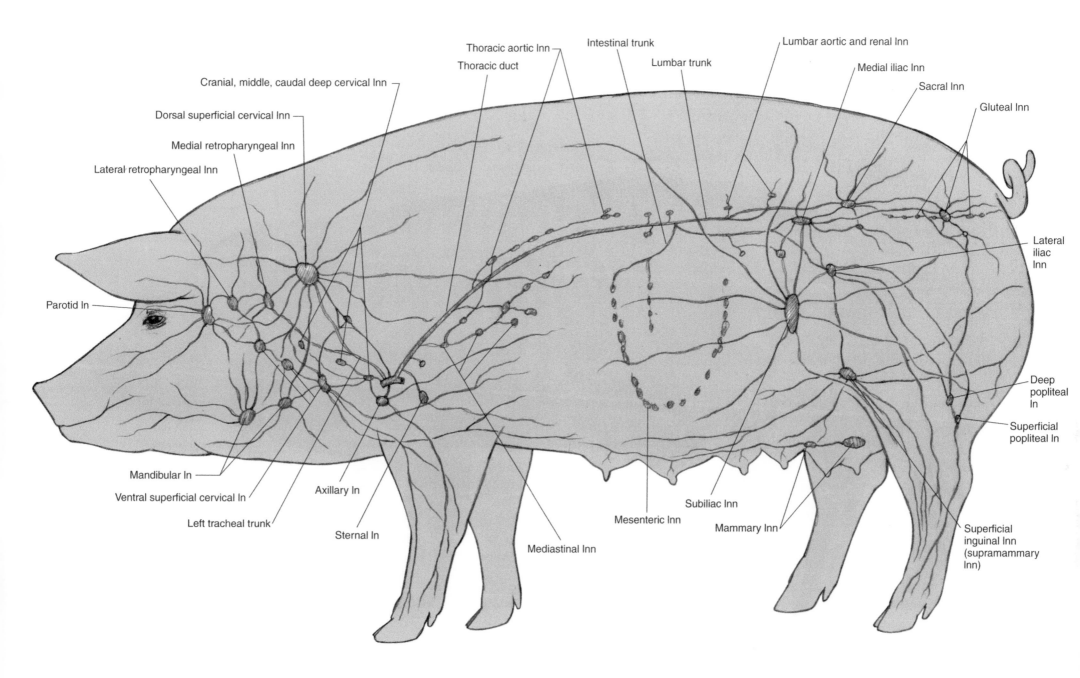

Thoracic aortic Inn

Intestinal trunk

Lumbar aortic and renal Inn

Thoracic duct

Lumbar trunk

Medial iliac Inn

Cranial, middle, caudal deep cervical Inn

Sacral Inn

Dorsal superficial cervical Inn

Gluteal Inn

Medial retropharyngeal Inn

Lateral retropharyngeal Inn

Lateral iliac Inn

Parotid In

Deep popliteal In

Superficial popliteal In

Mandibular In

Ventral superficial cervical In

Axillary In

Subiliac Inn

Left tracheal trunk

Sternal In

Mesenteric Inn

Mammary Inn

Mediastinal Inn

Superficial inguinal Inn (supramammary Inn)

121

PLATE 6.12 Lymph nodes and vessels of the sow. ln = lymph node

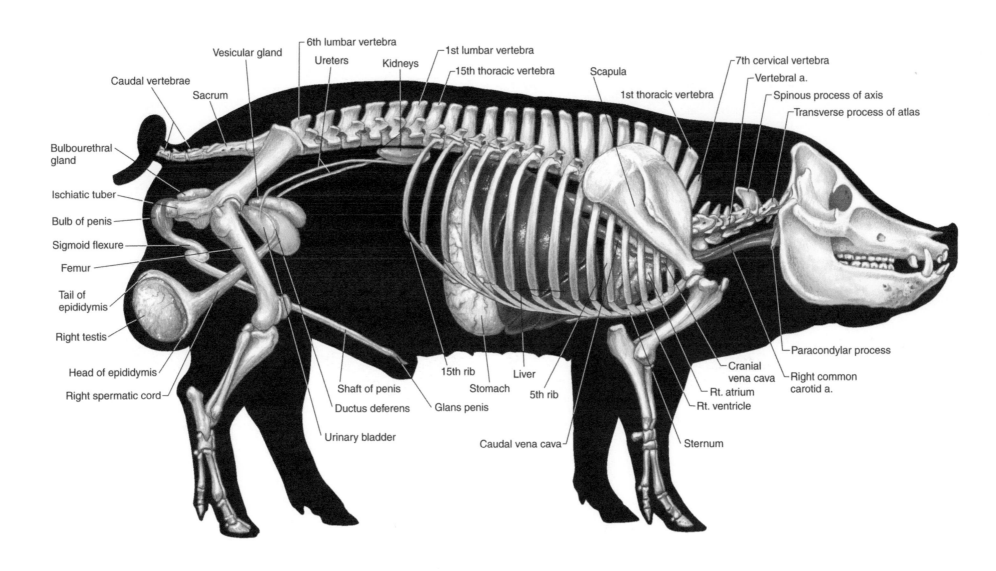

Caudal vertebrae

6th lumbar vertebra

Vesicular gland

Ureters

Kidneys

1st lumbar vertebra

15th thoracic vertebra

Scapula

7th cerviacl vertebra

1st thoracic vertebra

Vertebral a.

Sacrum

Spinous process of axis

Transverse process of atlas

Bulbourethral gland

Ischiatic tuber

Bulb of penis

Sigmoid flexure

Femur

Tail of epididymis

Right testis

Head of epididymis

Right spermatic cord

Shaft of penis

Ductus deferens

Glans penis

Urinary bladder

15th rib

Stomach

Liver

5th rib

Caudal vena cava

Cranial vena cava

Rt. atrium

Rt. ventricle

Sternum

Paracondylar process

Right common carotid a.

PLATE 6.13 Reproductive and urinary organs, stomach, liver, heart, and adjacent major vessels related to the skeleton of the boar. Lungs and intestines are removed. Right lateral view. a = artery

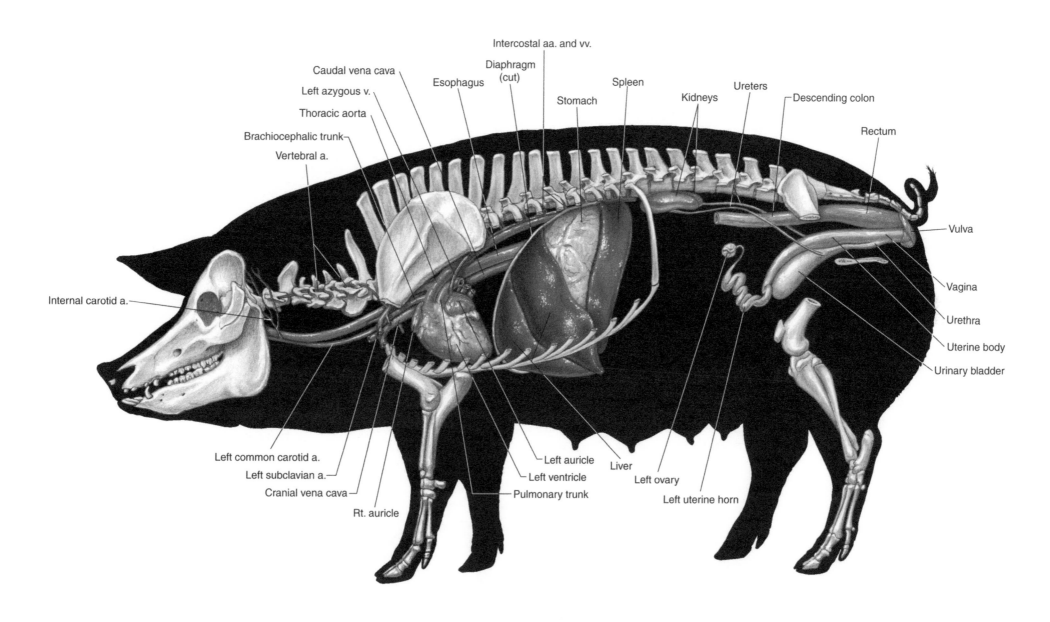

Intercostal aa. and vv.

Diaphragm (cut)

Caudal vena cava

Esophagus

Spleen

Left azygous v.

Stomach

Kidneys

Ureters

Descending colon

Thoracic aorta

Rectum

Brachiocephalic trunk

Vertebral a.

Internal carotid a.

Vulva

Vagina

Urethra

Uterine body

Urinary bladder

Left common carotid a.

Left auricle

Liver

Left subclavian a.

Left ventricle

Left ovary

Cranial vena cava

Pulmonary trunk

Left uterine horn

Rt. auricle

PLATE 6.14   Reproductive and urinary organs, abdominal viscera, spleen, heart, and adjacent major vessels of the sow. Lungs and intestines are removed. Left lateral view. v = vein, a = artery

123

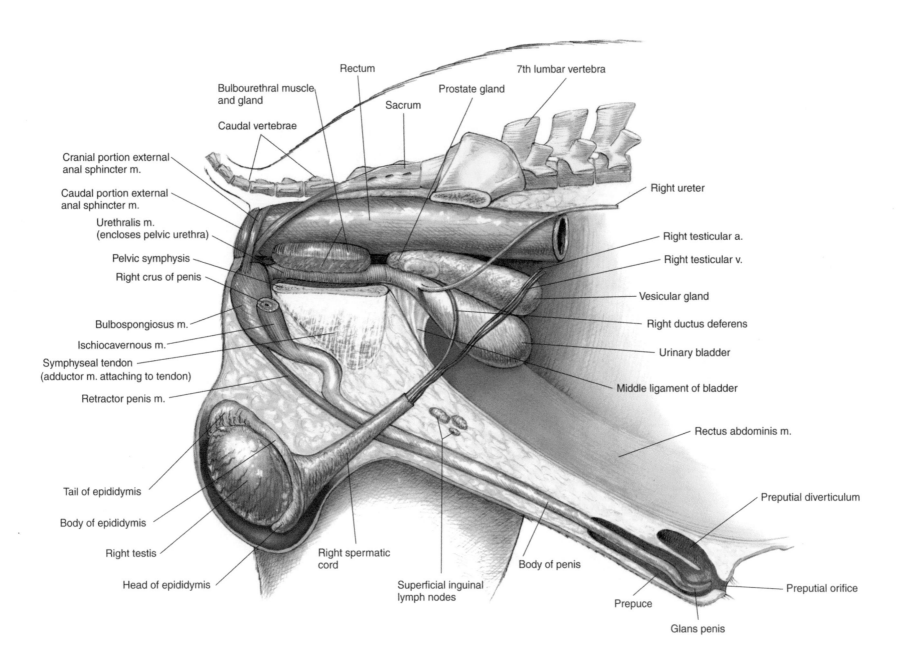

Rectum

Bulbourethral muscle
and gland

7th lumbar vertebra

Prostate gland

Caudal vertebrae

Sacrum

Cranial portion external
anal sphincter m.

Right ureter

Caudal portion external
anal sphincter m.

Urethralis m.
(encloses pelvic urethra)

Right testicular a.

Right testicular v.

Pelvic symphysis

Right crus of penis

Vesicular gland

Bulbospongiosus m.

Right ductus deferens

Ischiocavernous m.

Urinary bladder

Symphyseal tendon
(adductor m. attaching to tendon)

Middle ligament of bladder

Retractor penis m.

Rectus abdominis m.

Tail of epididymis

Preputial diverticulum

Body of epididymis

Right testis

Right spermatic
cord

Body of penis

Preputial orifice

Head of epididymis

Superficial inguinal
lymph nodes

Prepuce

Glans penis

PLATE 6.15 Relations of the reproductive organs of the boar. m = muscle, v = vein, a = artery

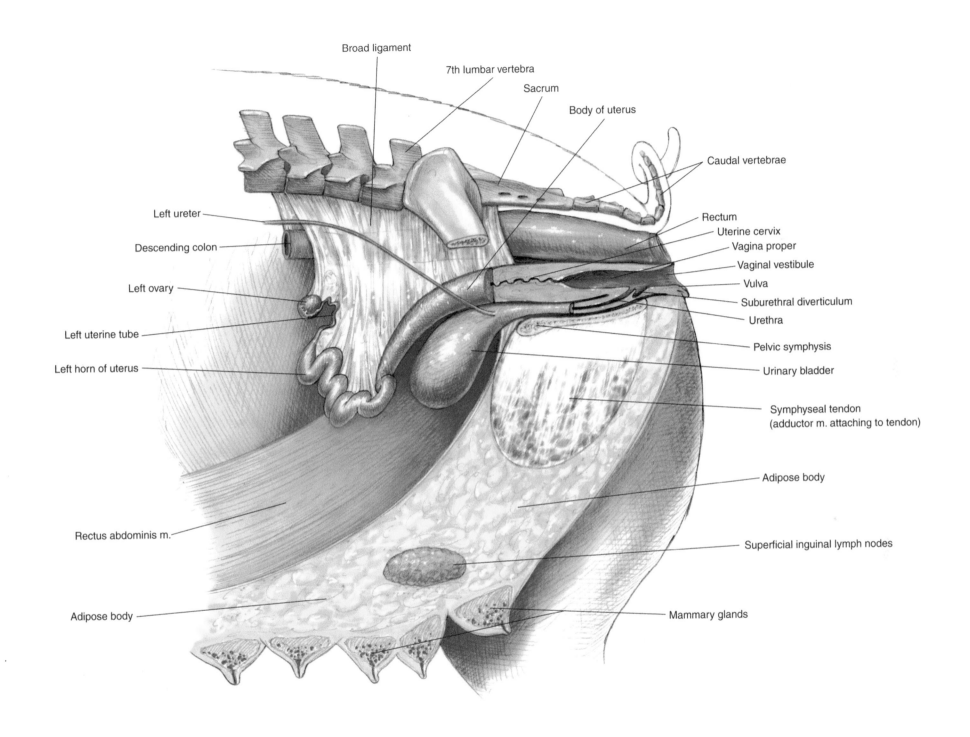

Broad ligament

7th lumbar vertebra

Sacrum

Body of uterus

Caudal vertebrae

Left ureter

Descending colon

Rectum

Uterine cervix

Vagina proper

Vaginal vestibule

Vulva

Left ovary

Suburethral diverticulum

Urethra

Left uterine tube

Pelvic symphysis

Left horn of uterus

Urinary bladder

Symphyseal tendon
(adductor m. attaching to tendon)

Adipose body

Rectus abdominis m.

Superficial inguinal lymph nodes

Adipose body

Mammary glands

125

PLATE 6.16 Relations of the reproductive organs of the sow.

SECTION 7 THE CHICKEN
(*Gallus gallus domesticus*)

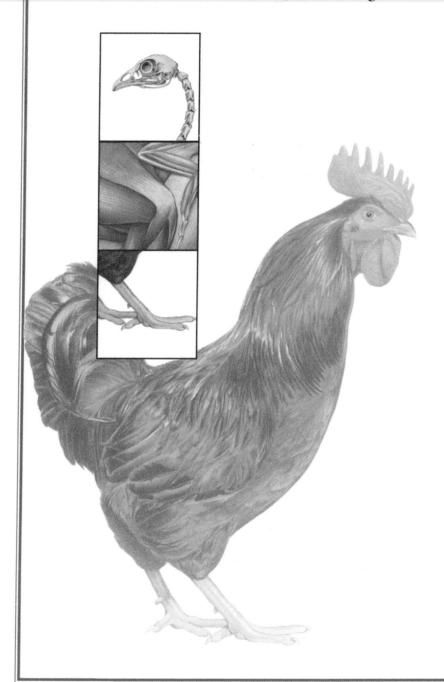

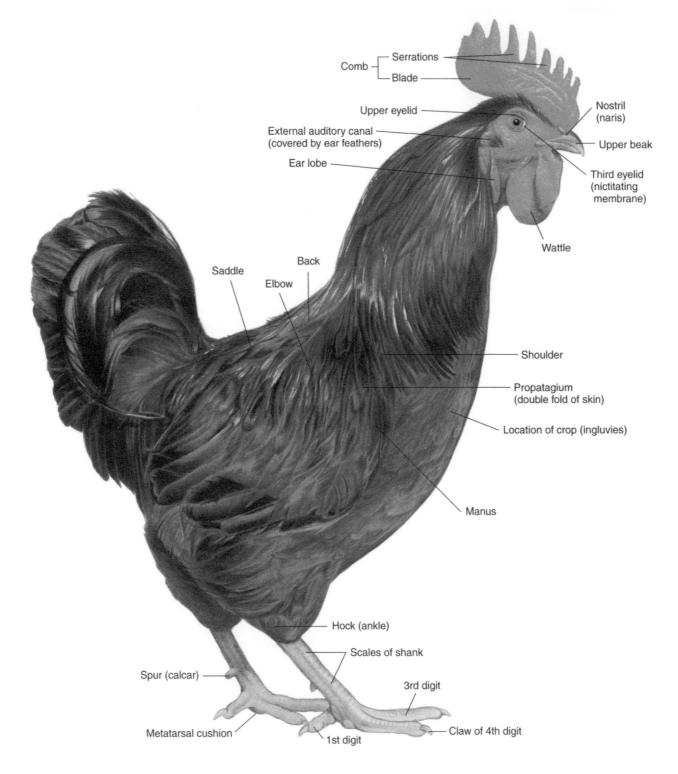

Comb — Serrations
Comb — Blade

Upper eyelid

External auditory canal
(covered by ear feathers)

Ear lobe

Nostril
(naris)

Upper beak

Third eyelid
(nictitating
membrane)

Wattle

Saddle

Back

Elbow

Shoulder

Propatagium
(double fold of skin)

Location of crop (ingluvies)

Manus

Hock (ankle)

Scales of shank

Spur (calcar)

3rd digit

Metatarsal cushion

1st digit

Claw of 4th digit

128

PLATE 7.1   Right lateral view of a rooster (cock).

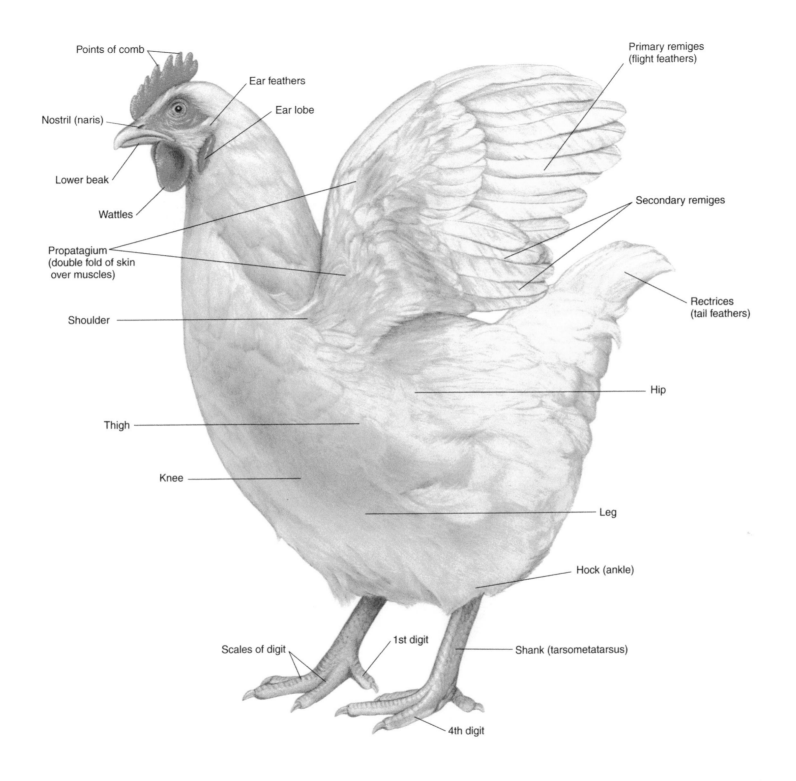

Points of comb

Ear feathers

Ear lobe

Nostril (naris)

Lower beak

Wattles

Propatagium
(double fold of skin
over muscles)

Shoulder

Thigh

Knee

Primary remiges
(flight feathers)

Secondary remiges

Rectrices
(tail feathers)

Hip

Leg

Hock (ankle)

Scales of digit

1st digit

Shank (tarsometatarsus)

4th digit

129

PLATE 7.2 Left lateral view of a hen. Patagiectomy (wing clipping), excision of part of
the propatagium (wing membrane), is performed on one wing to prevent flight.

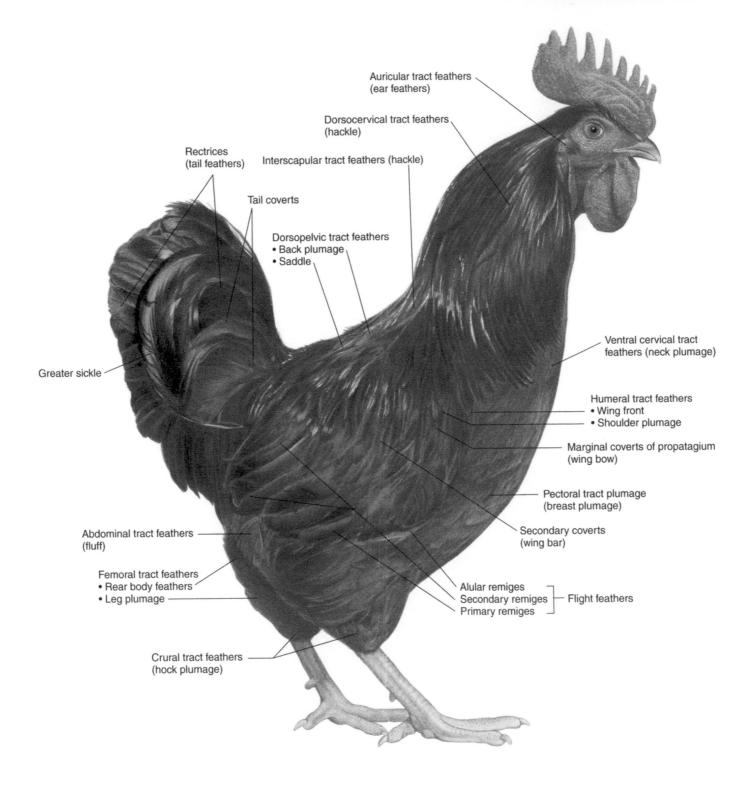

Auricular tract feathers
(ear feathers)

Dorsocervical tract feathers
(hackle)

Interscapular tract feathers (hackle)

Rectrices
(tail feathers)

Tail coverts

Dorsopelvic tract feathers
• Back plumage
• Saddle

Greater sickle

Ventral cervical tract
feathers (neck plumage)

Humeral tract feathers
• Wing front
• Shoulder plumage

Marginal coverts of propatagium
(wing bow)

Pectoral tract plumage
(breast plumage)

Abdominal tract feathers
(fluff)

Secondary coverts
(wing bar)

Femoral tract feathers
• Rear body feathers
• Leg plumage

Alular remiges
Secondary remiges
Primary remiges

Flight feathers

Crural tract feathers
(hock plumage)

PLATE 7.3 Feather coat of the rooster.

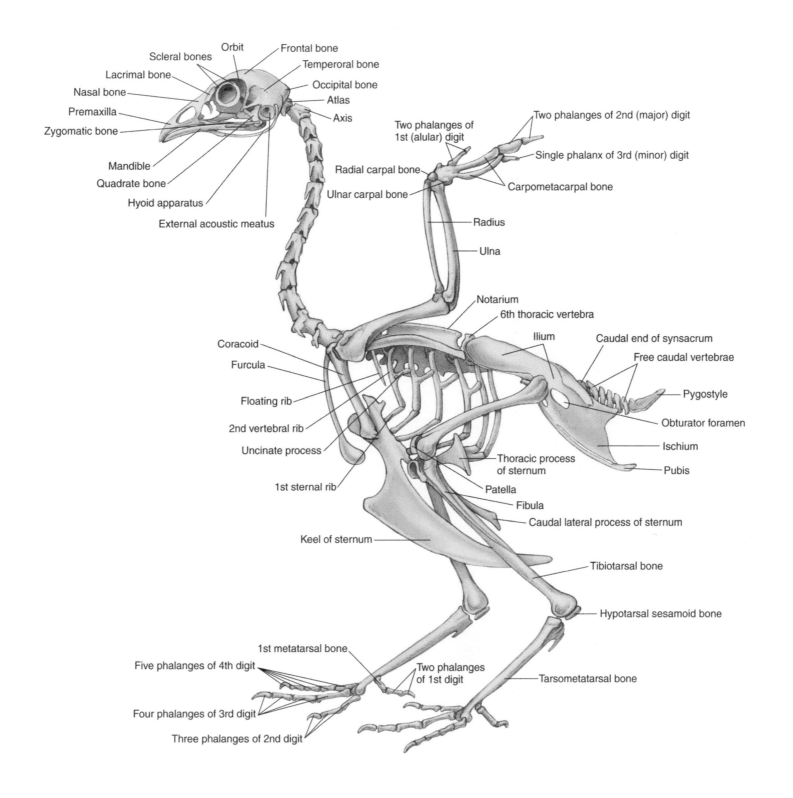

PLATE 7.4 Skeleton of the chicken. Left lateral view.

Orbit
Scleral bones
Frontal bone
Temperoral bone
Lacrimal bone
Occipital bone
Nasal bone
Atlas
Premaxilla
Axis
Zygomatic bone
Mandible
Quadrate bone
Hyoid apparatus
External acoustic meatus

Two phalanges of 1st (alular) digit
Two phalanges of 2nd (major) digit
Single phalanx of 3rd (minor) digit
Radial carpal bone
Ulnar carpal bone
Carpometacarpal bone
Radius
Ulna

Notarium
6th thoracic vertebra
Ilium
Caudal end of synsacrum
Coracoid
Free caudal vertebrae
Furcula
Floating rib
Pygostyle
2nd vertebral rib
Obturator foramen
Uncinate process
Ischium
Thoracic process of sternum
Pubis
1st sternal rib
Patella
Fibula
Caudal lateral process of sternum
Keel of sternum
Tibiotarsal bone
Hypotarsal sesamoid bone
1st metatarsal bone
Five phalanges of 4th digit
Two phalanges of 1st digit
Tarsometatarsal bone
Four phalanges of 3rd digit
Three phalanges of 2nd digit

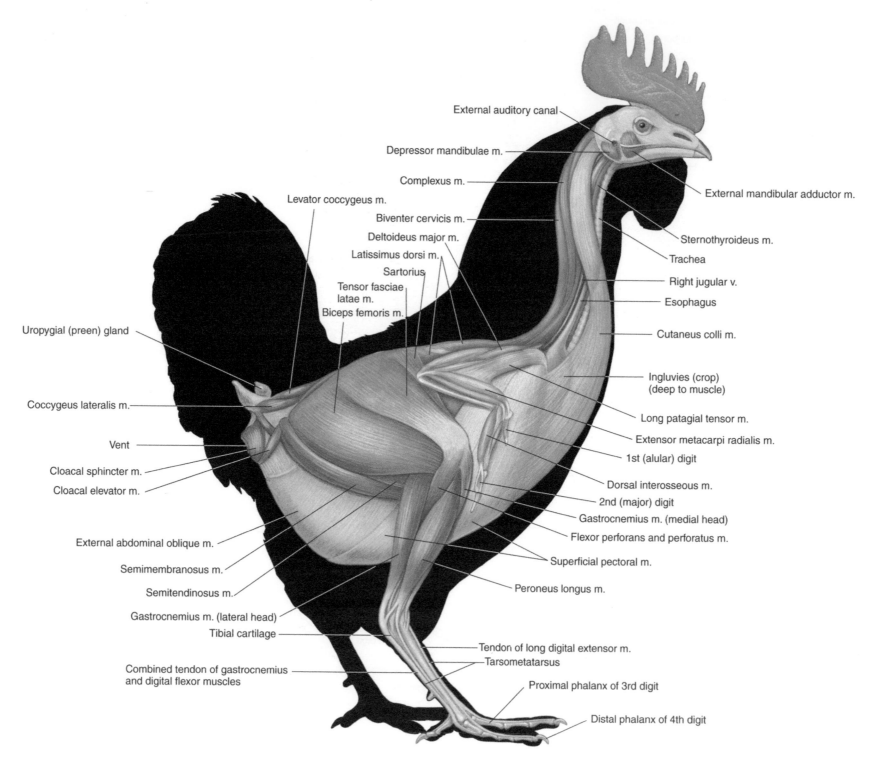

External auditory canal

Depressor mandibulae m.

Complexus m.

Levator coccygeus m.

Biventer cervicis m.

Deltoideus major m.

Latissimus dorsi m.

Sartorius

Tensor fasciae latae m.

Biceps femoris m.

External mandibular adductor m.

Sternothyroideus m.

Trachea

Right jugular v.

Esophagus

Cutaneus colli m.

Ingluvies (crop) (deep to muscle)

Uropygial (preen) gland

Long patagial tensor m.

Coccygeus lateralis m.

Extensor metacarpi radialis m.

Vent

1st (alular) digit

Cloacal sphincter m.

Dorsal interosseous m.

Cloacal elevator m.

2nd (major) digit

Gastrocnemius m. (medial head)

Flexor perforans and perforatus m.

External abdominal oblique m.

Superficial pectoral m.

Semimembranosus m.

Peroneus longus m.

Semitendinosus m.

Gastrocnemius m. (lateral head)

Tibial cartilage

Tendon of long digital extensor m.

Tarsometatarsus

Combined tendon of gastrocnemius and digital flexor muscles

Proximal phalanx of 3rd digit

Distal phalanx of 4th digit

132

PLATE 7.5 Superficial muscles of the rooster. Right lateral view. m = muscle, v = vein

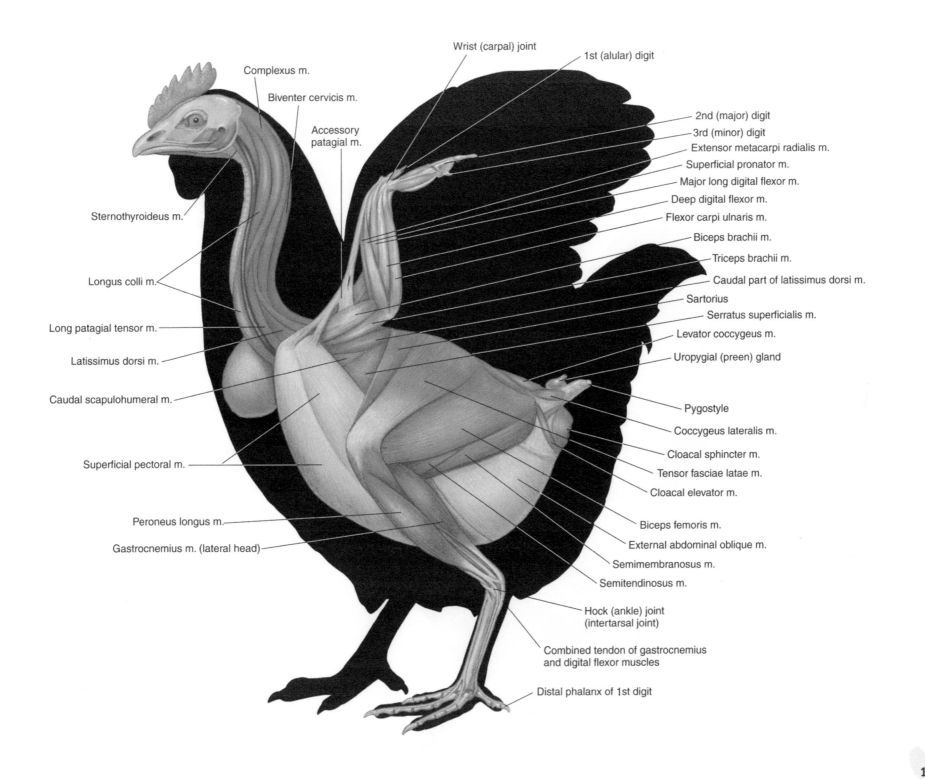

Complexus m.

Biventer cervicis m.

Accessory
patagial m.

Wrist (carpal) joint

1st (alular) digit

2nd (major) digit

3rd (minor) digit

Extensor metacarpi radialis m.

Superficial pronator m.

Major long digital flexor m.

Deep digital flexor m.

Flexor carpi ulnaris m.

Biceps brachii m.

Triceps brachii m.

Caudal part of latissimus dorsi m.

Sartorius

Serratus superficialis m.

Levator coccygeus m.

Uropygial (preen) gland

Pygostyle

Coccygeus lateralis m.

Cloacal sphincter m.

Tensor fasciae latae m.

Cloacal elevator m.

Biceps femoris m.

External abdominal oblique m.

Semimembranosus m.

Semitendinosus m.

Hock (ankle) joint
(intertarsal joint)

Combined tendon of gastrocnemius
and digital flexor muscles

Distal phalanx of 1st digit

Sternothyroideus m.

Longus colli m.

Long patagial tensor m.

Latissimus dorsi m.

Caudal scapulohumeral m.

Superficial pectoral m.

Peroneus longus m.

Gastrocnemius m. (lateral head)

133

PLATE 7.6 Superficial muscles of the hen. Left lateral view. m = muscle

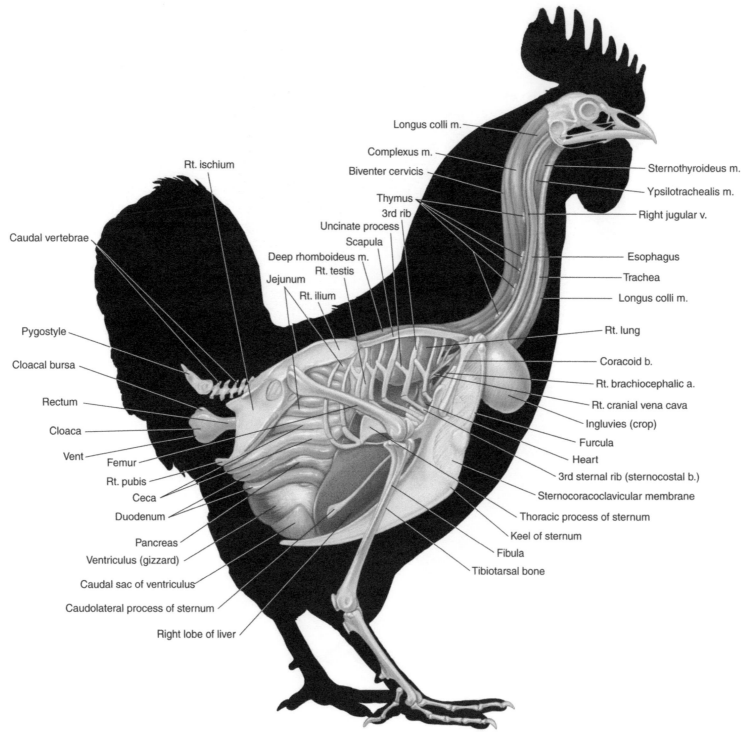

Longus colli m.

Complexus m.

Biventer cervicis

Thymus

3rd rib

Uncinate process

Scapula

Deep rhomboideus m.

Rt. testis

Jejunum

Rt. ilium

Rt. ischium

Caudal vertebrae

Pygostyle

Cloacal bursa

Rectum

Cloaca

Vent

Femur

Rt. pubis

Ceca

Duodenum

Pancreas

Ventriculus (gizzard)

Caudal sac of ventriculus

Caudolateral process of sternum

Right lobe of liver

Sternothyroideus m.

Ypsilotrachealis m.

Right jugular v.

Esophagus

Trachea

Longus colli m.

Rt. lung

Coracoid b.

Rt. brachiocephalic a.

Rt. cranial vena cava

Ingluvies (crop)

Furcula

Heart

3rd sternal rib (sternocostal b.)

Sternocoracoclavicular membrane

Thoracic process of sternum

Keel of sternum

Fibula

Tibiotarsal bone

PLATE 7.7 Relations of *in situ* viscera to the skeleton and cervical muscles of the rooster. Right lateral view. m = muscle, b = bone, a = artery, v = vein

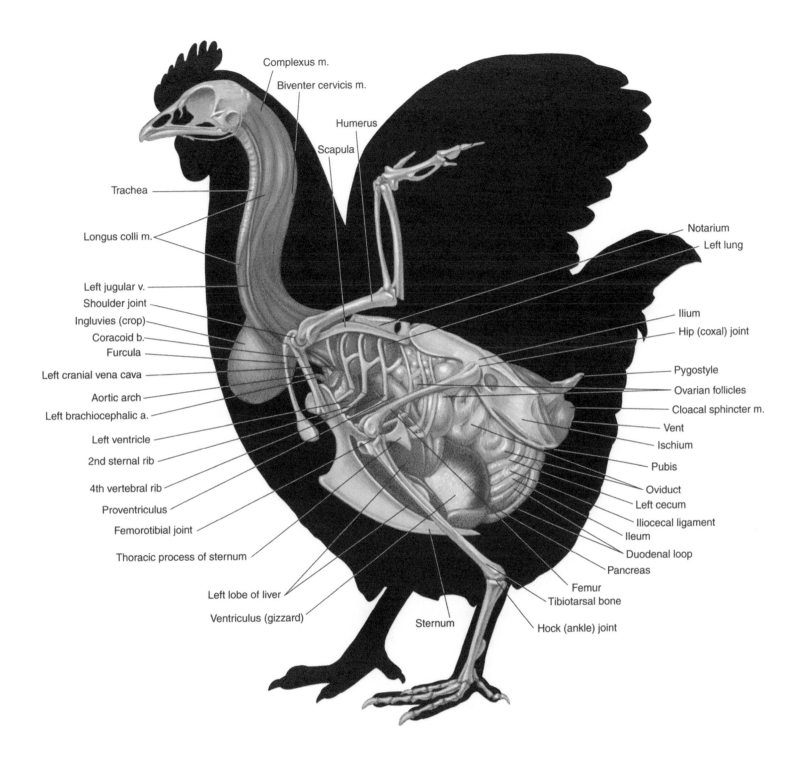

Complexus m.

Biventer cervicis m.

Humerus

Scapula

Trachea

Longus colli m.

Notarium

Left lung

Left jugular v.

Shoulder joint

Ingluvies (crop)

Coracoid b.

Furcula

Left cranial vena cava

Aortic arch

Left brachiocephalic a.

Left ventricle

2nd sternal rib

4th vertebral rib

Proventriculus

Femorotibial joint

Thoracic process of sternum

Left lobe of liver

Ventriculus (gizzard)

Sternum

Ilium

Hip (coxal) joint

Pygostyle

Ovarian follicles

Cloacal sphincter m.

Vent

Ischium

Pubis

Oviduct

Left cecum

Iliocecal ligament

Ileum

Duodenal loop

Pancreas

Femur

Tibiotarsal bone

Hock (ankle) joint

135

PLATE 7.8 Relations of *in situ* viscera and blood vessels to the skeleton and cervical
muscles of the hen. Left lateral view. m = muscle, v = vein, b = bone, a = artery

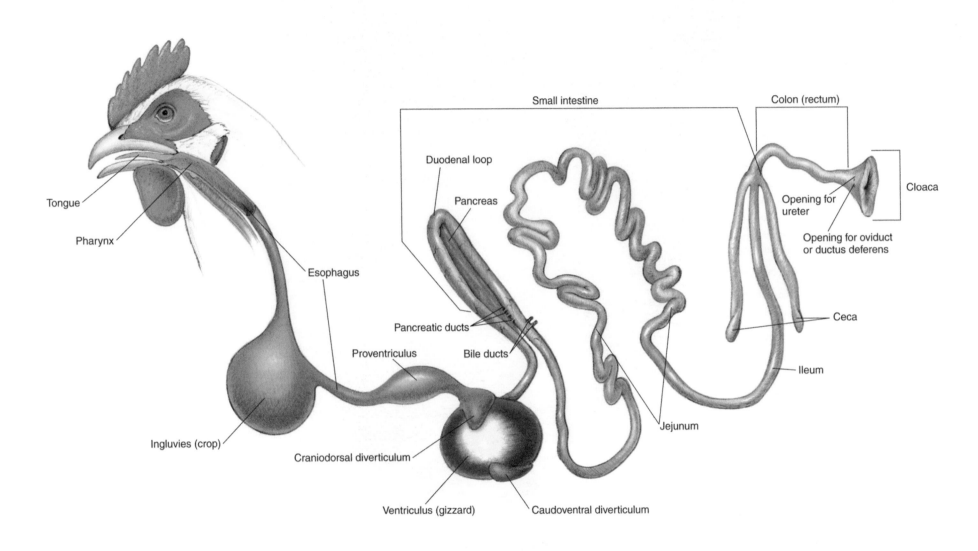

Tongue

Pharynx

Esophagus

Ingluvies (crop)

Proventriculus

Craniodorsal diverticulum

Ventriculus (gizzard)

Caudoventral diverticulum

Small intestine

Duodenal loop

Pancreas

Pancreatic ducts

Bile ducts

Jejunum

Colon (rectum)

Opening for ureter

Opening for oviduct or ductus deferens

Cloaca

Ceca

Ileum

PLATE 7.9   Isolated gastrointestinal tract of the chicken.

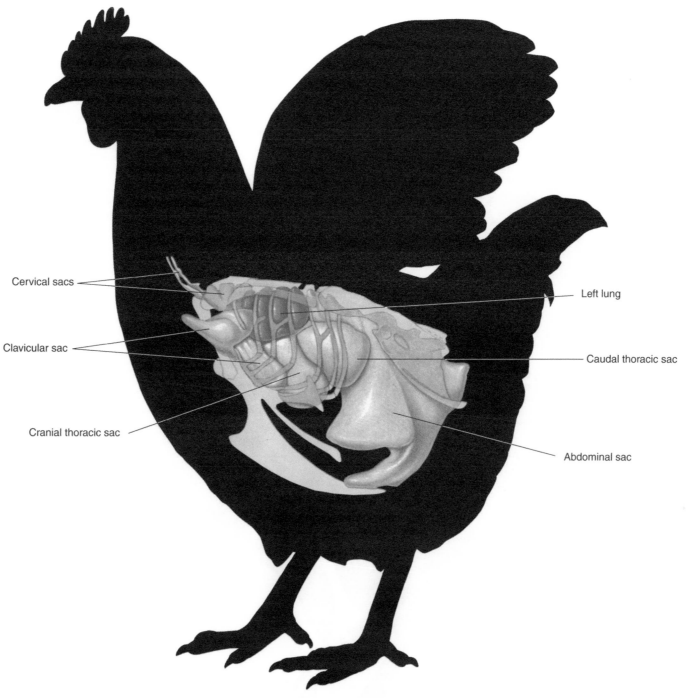

Cervical sacs

Clavicular sac

Cranial thoracic sac

Left lung

Caudal thoracic sac

Abdominal sac

PLATE 7.10   Air sacs and lungs of the chicken. Left lateral view. There is a total of eleven air sacs named according to location: abdominal, caudal thoracic, cranial thoracic, axillary, clavicular, and cervical. All are paired except the single clavicular sac. With the exception of the thoracic sacs, all provide communication between a bronchus and the interior of some of the pneumatic (air-containing) bones.

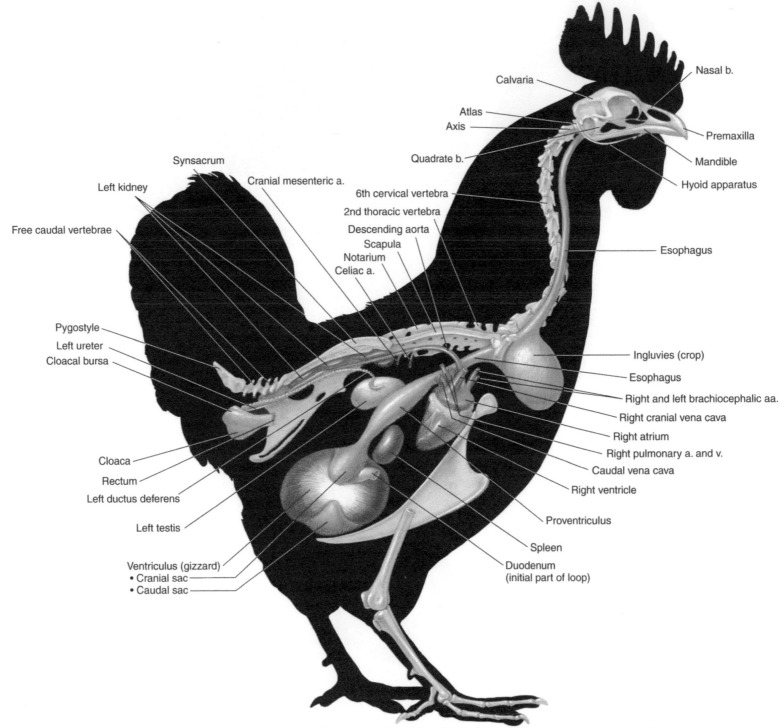

Calvaria

Nasal b.

Atlas

Axis

Quadrate b.

Premaxilla

Mandible

Hyoid apparatus

Synsacrum

Cranial mesenteric a.

Left kidney

6th cervical vertebra

2nd thoracic vertebra

Descending aorta

Scapula

Notarium

Celiac a.

Esophagus

Free caudal vertebrae

Pygostyle

Left ureter

Cloacal bursa

Ingluvies (crop)

Esophagus

Right and left brachiocephalic aa.

Right cranial vena cava

Right atrium

Right pulmonary a. and v.

Caudal vena cava

Right ventricle

Cloaca

Rectum

Left ductus deferens

Left testis

Proventriculus

Spleen

Duodenum
(initial part of loop)

Ventriculus (gizzard)
• Cranial sac
• Caudal sac

138

PLATE 7.11 *In situ* viscera, major blood vessels, and axial skeleton of the rooster. Intestines, liver, and lungs are removed. Right lateral view. b = bone, a = artery, v = vein

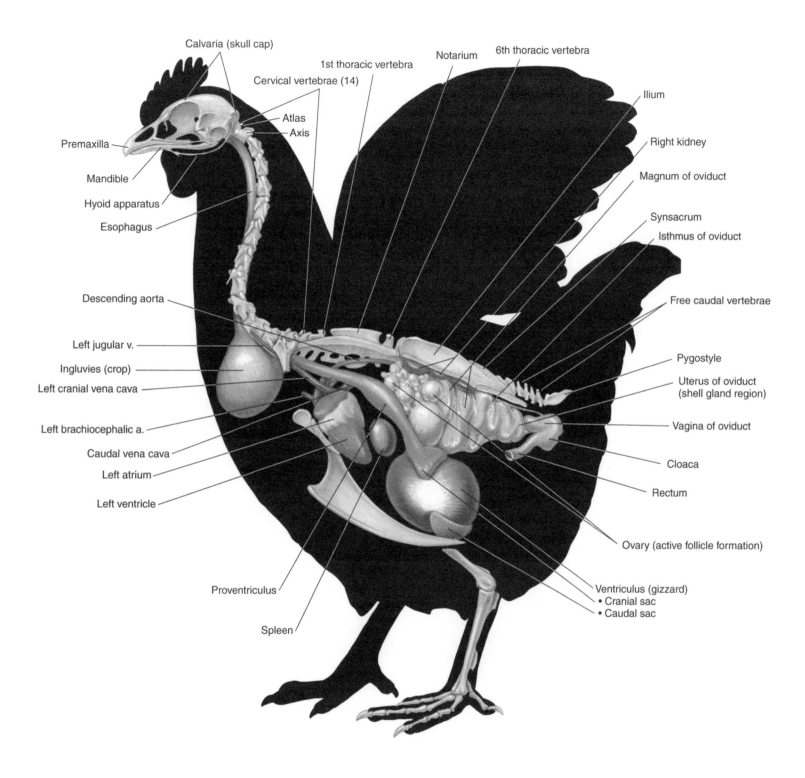

PLATE 7.12 *In situ* viscera, major blood vessels, and axial skeleton of the hen. Intestines, liver, and lungs are removed. Left lateral view. v = vein, a = artery

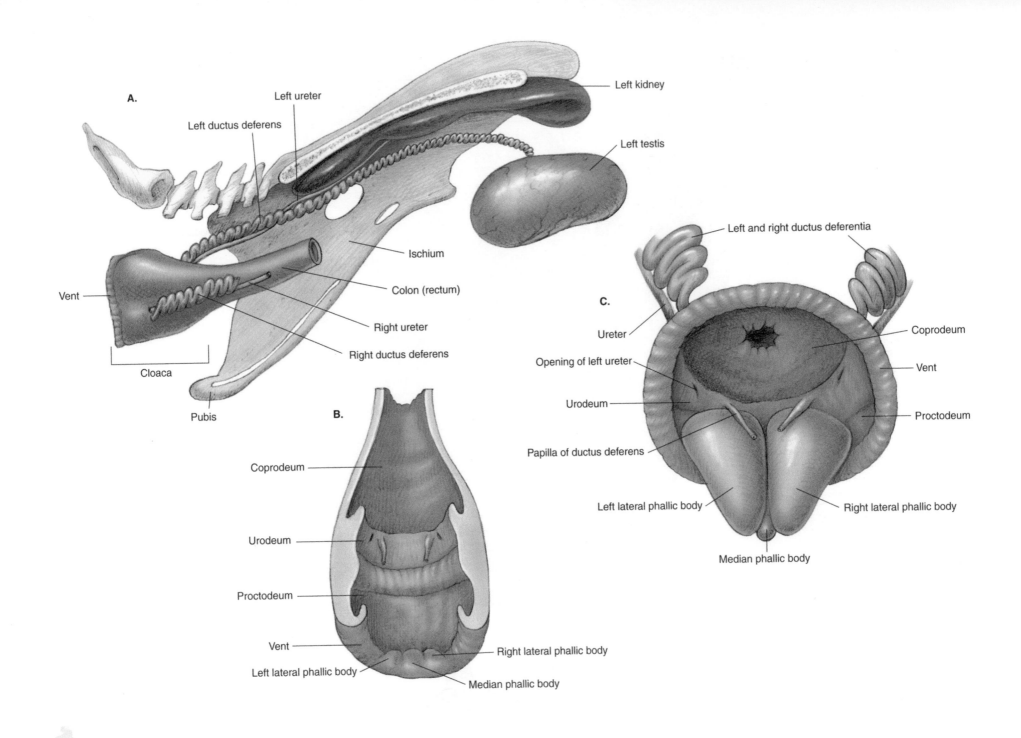

A.

Left ureter

Left ductus deferens

Left kidney

Left testis

Ischium

Vent

Colon (rectum)

Right ureter

Right ductus deferens

Cloaca

Pubis

B.

Coprodeum

Urodeum

Proctodeum

Vent

Left lateral phallic body

Right lateral phallic body

Median phallic body

C.

Left and right ductus deferentia

Ureter

Opening of left ureter

Urodeum

Papilla of ductus deferens

Coprodeum

Vent

Proctodeum

Left lateral phallic body

Right lateral phallic body

Median phallic body

PLATE 7. 13 **A.** Reproductive and urinary organs of the rooster. Right lateral view. **B.** Cloaca of the rooster. Dorsal view. **C.** Erect copulatory apparatus. Caudodorsal view.

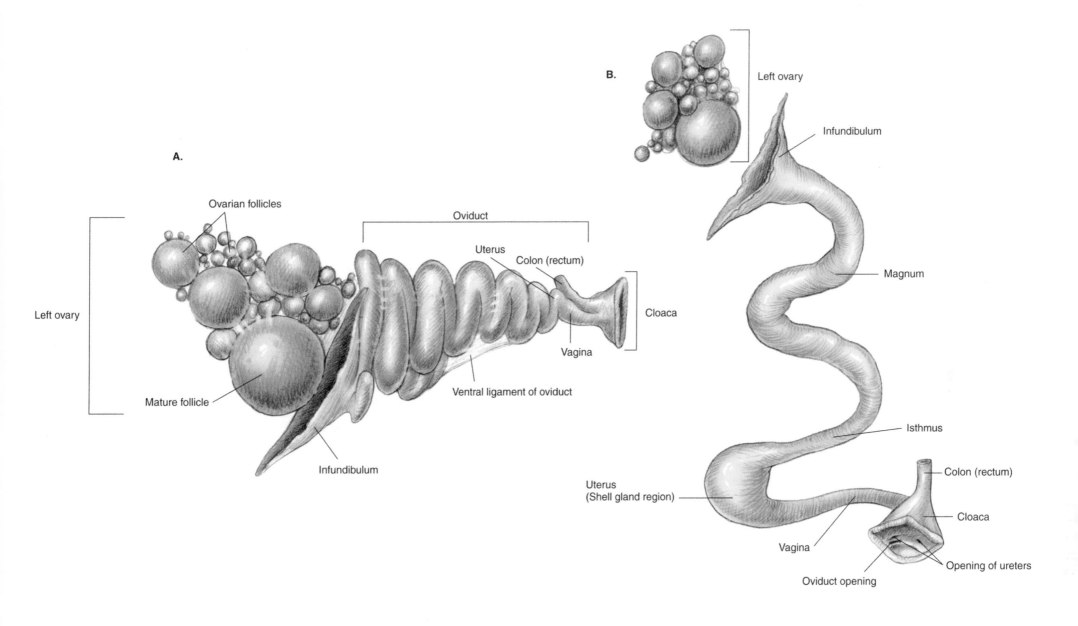

A.

Ovarian follicles

Oviduct

Uterus

Colon (rectum)

Cloaca

Left ovary

Vagina

Mature follicle

Ventral ligament of oviduct

Infundibulum

B.

Left ovary

Infundibulum

Magnum

Isthmus

Uterus
(Shell gland region)

Colon (rectum)

Cloaca

Vagina

Opening of ureters

Oviduct opening

141

PLATE 7.14 **A.** Isolated reproductive organs of the hen. Left lateral view.
B. Diagrammatic representation of the reproductive organs of the hen.

BIBLIOGRAPHY

Ashdown PR, Done SH. Color Atlas of Veterinary Anatomy—The Ruminants. London: Bailliere Tindall, 1984.

Ashdown PR, Done SH. Color Atlas of Veterinary Anatomy—The Horse. London: Bailliere Tindall, 1987.

Budras K-D, Sack WO, Rock S. Anatomy of the Horse—An Illustrated Text. London: Mosby-Wolfe, 1994.

Chamberlain F. Atlas of Avian Anatomy. East Lansing, Michigan: State College Press, 1943.

Clayton HM, Flood PF. Color Atlas of Large Animal Applied Anatomy. London: Mosby-Wolfe, 1996.

de Lahunta A, Habel RE. Applied Veterinary Anatomy. Philadelphia: WB Saunders, 1986.

Dyce KM, Sack WO, Wensing GJG. Textbook of Veterinary Anatomy. Philadelphia: WB Saunders, 1987.

Ellenberger W. Leisering's Atlas of Anatomy, Vol 1. Chicago: Alexander Eger, 1908.

Ellenberger W, Dittrich H, Baum HM. An Atlas of Animal Anatomy. London: Dover, 1949.

Ellenberger W, Baum HM. Handbuch der Vergleichenden Anatomie der Haustiere. 18th ed. Berlin: Springer, 1977.

Fowler ME. Medicine and Surgery of South American Camelids: Llama, Alpaca, Vicuna, Guanaco. Ames, IA: Iowa State University Press, 1995.

Garrett PD. Guide to Ruminant Anatomy Based on the Dissection of the Goat. Ames, IA: Iowa State University Press, 1988.

Gertty R. Sisson and Grossman's The Anatomy of the Domestic Animals, 5th ed, Vols I and II. Philadelphia: WB Saunders, 1975.

Goshal NG, Koch T, Popesko P. The Venous Drainage of the Domestic Animals. Philadelphia: WB Saunders, 1981.

Harvey EB, Kaiser HE, Rosenberg LE. An Atlas of the Domestic Turkey. United States Atomic Energy Commission, 1948.

Kainer RA. Functional anatomy of equine locomotor organs. In: Stashak T, ed. Adams' Lameness in Horses. 5th ed. Philadelphia: Lippincott Williams & Wilkins, 1999.

Kainer RA, McCracken TO. Horse Anatomy—A Coloring Atlas. 2nd ed. Loveland, CO: Alpine Publications, 1998.

McLeod WM, Trotter DM, Lumb JW. Avian Anatomy. Minneapolis: Burgess Publishing Co, 1964.

The Meat Buyers Guide. National Association of Meat Purveyors, McLean, VA, 1992.

Moreng RE, Avens JS. Poultry Science and Production. Prospect Heights, IL: Waveland Press, 1981.

Nickel R, Schummer A, Seiferle E, et al. The Locomotor System of the Domestic Animals, Vol 1. Berlin-Hamburg: Paul Parey, 1986.

Nickel R, Schummer A, Seiferle E. Nervensystem. Sinnesorgane und Endokrine Drusen, Vol 4. Berlin-Hamburg: Paul Parey, 1992.

Nickel R, Schummer A, Seiferle E. Anatomy of the Domestic Birds, Vol 5. Berlin-Hamburg: Paul Parey, 1977.

Pfizer Animal Health Group. Anatomical Atlas. New York: Pfizer Corporation, 1976.

Popesko P. Atlas of Topographic Anatomy of the Domestic Animals. Philadelphia: WB Saunders, 1979.

Sack WO, Habel RE. Rooney's Guide to the Dissection of the Horse. Ithaca, NY: Veterinary Textbooks, 1977.

Sack WO, Horowitz A. Essentials of Pig Anatomy & Atlas of Musculoskeletal Anatomy of the Pig. Ithaca, NY: Veterinary Textbooks, 1982.

Schummer A, Nickel R, Sack WO. The Viscera of the Domestic Animals, Vol 2. Berlin-Hamburg: Paul Parey, 1979.

Schummer A, Wilkins H, Vollmerhaus B, Habermehl K-H. The Circulatory System, the Skin, and the Cutaneous Organs of the Domestic Animals, Vol 3. Berlin-Hamburg: Paul Parey, 1981.

Senger PL. Pathways to Pregnancy and Parturition. Pullman, WA: Senger, 1997.

Shively MJ. Veterinary Anatomy—Basic, Comparative and Clinical. College Station, TX: Texas A & M University, 1984.

Smallwood JE. A Guided Tour of Veterinary Anatomy. Philadelphia: WB Saunders, 1992.

INDEX

References to the various animals described in this atlas are indicated by the following letters preceding page numbers: **H,** horse; **O,** ox; **S,** sheep; **G,** goat; **L,** llama and alpaca; **Sw,** swine; **C,** chicken.

A

Abdomen, **L** 90; **Sw** 111
Abdominal tunic, **O** 37
Abomasum, **O** 38, 42, 43, 45; **S** 60, 61, 64, 65; **G** 80, 81, 84
Adipose body, **Sw** 125
Air sacs, **C** 137
Ankle, **H** 2 (fetlock); **C** 128, 129 (hock)
Antebrachium, **H** 2; **O** 33; **G** 72; **L** 90
Anus, **H** 13, 20, 22, 23; **O** 41, 45, 46, 47; **S** 67; **G** 85, 86, 87; **L** 106, 107; **Sw** 117
Aorta. *See* Artery or Arteries
Arm, **H** 2; **O** 32, 33; **S** 54; **G** 72; **L** 90
Artery or Arteries
    aorta, **H** 24, 25; **O** 44, 45, 49; **S** 64, 64; **G** 84, 85, 87; **L** 104, 105; **Sw** 123; **C** 135, 138, 139
    artery of the lateral sinus, **G** 87
    axillary, **H** 25, 49
    bicarotid trunk, **S** 65; **G** 85
    brachial, **H** 25; **O** 49
    brachiocephalic trunk, **H** 21, 25; **O** 45, 49; **S** 65; **L** 104, 105; **Sw** 123
    bronchoesophageal, **O** 49
    caudal auricular, **H** 25; **O** 49; **G** 82
    caudal epigastric, **H** 25; **O** 49; **G** 85, 87
    caudal femoral, **H** 25; **O** 49
    caudal gluteal, **H** 25; **O** 49; **G** 87
    caudal interosseous, **O** 49
    caudal mammary, **O** 49; **G** 87
    caudal meningeal, **G** 82
    caudal mesenteric, **H** 25; **O** 49
    caudal superficial epigastric, **G** 87
    caudal tibial, **H** 25; **O** 49
    celiac, **H** 25; **O** 49; **C** 138
    collateral ulnar, **H** 25; **O** 49
    common carotid, **H** 25; **O** 44, 45, 49; **S** 62, 64, 65; **G** 82, 84, 85; **L** 101, 104, 105; **Sw** 122, 123
    common interosseous, **H** 20, 21, 25; **O** 44, 45, 59; **S** 62, 64, 65; **G** 82, 84, 85
    condylar, **G** 82
    cornual, **G** 80, 82
    costocervical trunk, **H** 25
    cranial epigastric, **H** 25; **O** 49
    cranial gluteal, **H** 25; **O** 49
    cranial interosseous, **O** 49
    cranial mammary, **O** 49; **G** 87
    cranial mesenteric, **H** 25; **O** 49; **C** 138
    cranial tibial, **H** 25; **O** 49
    deep cervical, **H** 25; **O** 49
    deep circumflex iliac, **H** 25; **O** 49
    deep femoral, **H** 25; **O** 49; **G** 85, 87
    descending genicular, **H** 25
    digital, **H** 25; **G** 78; **L** 96
    distal perforating branch, **H** 25
    dorsal, **H** 25; **O** 49
    dorsal common digital, **O** 49
    dorsal metacarpal III, **O** 49
    dorsal metatarsal III, **O** 49
    dorsal nasal, **G** 82
    dorsal pedal, **H** 25; **O** 49
    dorsal proper digital, **O** 49
    ethmoid, **G** 82

B

Back, **H** 2; **O** 32; **S** 54; **G** 72; **L** 90; **Sw** 110, 111; **C** 128, 130

Barrel, **H** 3; **O** 33; **L** 90

Beak, **C** 128, 129

Beard, **G** 72

Body regions, **H** 4; **O** 34; **G** 74; **L** 91

    dorsal vertebral regions, **O** 38; **S** 55; **G** 73; **L** 91

    perineal region, **O** 33

Bone(s)

    atlas, **H** 5, 12, 14, 20; **O** 35, 39, 44, 45; **S** 57, 61, 64; **G** 75, 81, 83; **L** 93, 97, 99; **Sw** 113, 118, 122; **C** 131, 138, 139

    axis, **H** 5, 14, 20; **O** 35, 45; **S** 57; **G** 75, 83; **L** 93, 99; **Sw** 113, 118, 122; **C** 131, 138, 139

    basihyoid, **H** 14; **O** 40; **G** 83; **L** 99; **Sw** 118

    calcaneus, **H** 5; **O** 35; **S** 57; **G** 75; **L** 93; **Sw** 113

        calcaneal tuber, **H** 5; **O** 35; **S** 57; **G** 73, 75; **L** 91; **Sw** 110, 113

    calvaria (skull cap), **C** 131, 138, 139

    cannon, **H** 5. *See* Third metacarpal/metatarsal

    carpal, **H** 5; **O** 35; **S** 57; **G** 75; **L** 93; **Sw** 113; **C** 131

    carpometacarpal, **C** 131

    coffin, **H** 5

    coracoid, **C** 131, 134

    ethmoid, **H** 14; **G** 83; **L** 99; **Sw** 118

    femur, **H** 5; **O** 35, 39; **S** 57, 64; **G** 75; **L** 93, 104; **Sw** 113, 122; **C** 131, 134, 135

        greater trochanter, **H** 5; **O** 35, 38, 39; **S** 57, 60; **G** 75, 80; **L** 93; **Sw** 113

    fibula, **H** 5; **Sw** 113; **C** 131, 134

    frontal, **H** 5, 14; **O** 35, 40; **S** 57, 60; **G** 75, 80, 82, 83, 84; **L** 93, 99, 102; **Sw** 113, 118, 119; **C** 131

        cornual process, **S** 57, 60; **G** 80

    furcula, **C** 131, 134, 135

    humerus, **H** 5, 8; **O** 35, 39; **S** 57, 64; **G** 75; **L** 93, 104; **Sw** 113; **C** 131, 135

        deltoid tuberosity, **H** 5

        greater tubercle, **H** 5; **O** 32, 35; **S** 57; **G** 73, 75; **L** 93; **Sw** 111, 113

        lateral epicondyle, **H** 5; **G** 75; **L** 93

    hyoid apparatus, **H** 13; **C** 131

    ilium, **H** 5; **O** 35; **S** 57, 64; **G** 75; **L** 93, 104; **Sw** 113, 117, 122; **C** 131, 134, 135, 136, 139

        body, **H** 5; **O** 35; **S** 57; **G** 75; **L** 93

        coxal tuber, **H** 5, 7, 13; **O** 32, 35, 37, 39; **S** 57, 58; **G** 73, 75, 76; **L** 93, 95; **Sw** 111, 113, 115, 117

        sacral tuber, **H** 5

        wing, **H** 5; **O** 35; **S** 57; **G** 75

    incisive, **H** 5, 14; **O** 35; **S** 57, 60; **G** 75, 80, 82, 84; **L** 93, 102; **Sw** 113, 119

    interparietal, **L** 102

    ischium, **H** 5; **O** 35, 44; **S** 57; **G** 75; **L** 93; **Sw** 113, 117; **C** 131, 134, 135, 140

        ischiatic tuber, **H** 5, 13; **O** 32, 35, 39; **S** 57, 61, 64; **G** 75, 76; **L** 93, 95; **Sw** 113, 117, 122

    lacrimal, **H** 5; **O** 35; **S** 57; **G** 75; **L** 93, 102; **Sw** 113, 119; **C** 131

    mandible, **H** 5, 15; **O** 35, 40; **S** 57, 60; **G** 75, 80, 82, 83, 84; **L** 93, 99, 102; **Sw** 113, 118, 119; **C** 131, 138, 139

        coronoid process, **O** 44; **G** 84; **L** 93

        mental foramen (foramina), **H** 5, 15; **O** 35; **S** 57; **G** 75; **L** 102; **Sw** 113, 119

    maxilla, **H** 5, 12, 15; **O** 35; **S** 57, 60; **G** 75, 82, 84; **L** 93, 102; **Sw** 113, 119

        facial crest, **H** 3, 5

        facial tuber, **O** 35

        infraorbital foramen, **H** 5; **O** 35; **S** 57; **G** 75; **L** 93, 102; **Sw** 113, 119

    metacarpal

        fifth, **O** 35; **S** 57; **G** 75; **Sw** 113

        fourth, **H** 5; **O** 35; **S** 57; **G** 75; **L** 93; **Sw** 113

        second, **H** 5; **O** 35; **Sw** 113;

        third, **H** 5; **O** 35; **S** 57; **G** 75; **L** 93; **Sw** 113

    metacarpal tuberosity, **H** 5, 10

    metatarsal

        fifth, **Sw** 113

        fourth, **H** 5; **O** 35; **S** 57; **G** 75; **L** 93; **Sw** 113

        second, **H** 5; **O** 35; **Sw** 113

        third, **H** 5; **O** 35; **S** 57; **G** 75; **L** 93; **Sw** 113

    nasal, **H** 5, 12, 14; **O** 35; **S** 57; **G** 75, 80, 82, 83; **L** 99, 102; **Sw** 113, 118, 119; **C** 131, 138

    navicular, **H** 8

Bone(s)—*Continued*

notarium, **C** 131, 138, 139

occipital, **H** 5, 14; **O** 35, 40; **S** 57, 60; **G** 75, 82, 83; **L** 93, 99, 102; **Sw** 113, 118, 119; **C** 131

nuchal crest, **O** 35

palatine, **H** 14; **O** 35

paracondylar process, **L** 102; **Sw** 122

parietal, **H** 5, 14; **O** 35; **S** 27; **G** 75; **G** 75, 83; **L** 93, 99, 102; **Sw** 119

patella, **H** 5, 11; **O** 35; **S** 57; **G** 75; **L** 93; **Sw** 113; **C** 131

phalanges, **H** 5, 8, 9; **O** 35; **S** 57; **G** 75, 79; **L** 93; **Sw** 113; **C** 131, 132, 133

premaxilla, **C** 131, 138, 139

presphenoid, **O** 40

pubis, **H** 5; **O** 35; **S** 57; **G** 75; **L** 93; **Sw** 113, 117; **C** 131, 133, 134, 135, 140

pygostyle, **C** 131, 133, 134, 135, 138, 139

quadrate, **C** 131, 138

radius, **H** 5; **O** 35; **S** 57; **G** 75; **L** 93; **Sw** 113; **C** 131

trochlea, **O** 35

ribs, **H** 5, 20; **O** 35, 38, 39, 44; **S** 57, 64, 64; **G** 75, 81, 84, 85; **L** 93, 104; **Sw** 113, 122; **C** 131, 134, 135

rib margin, **G** 73; **L** 91

uncinate process, **C** 131, 134

rostral,**Sw** 113, 118, 119

sacrum, **H** 5, 20, 22, 25; **O** 35, 44, 46, 47; **S** 57, 64, 66, 67; **G** 75, 84, 86; **L** 93, 106, 107; **Sw** 113, 117, 122, 124, 125

scapula, **H** 3, 5; **O** 35; **S** 57; **G** 75; **L** 93; **Sw** 113, 122; **C** 131, 134, 135

acromion, **O** 35, 39; **S** 57; **G** 75, 81; **L** 93

scapular cartilage, **H** 5; **O** 35, 38; **S** 57; **G** 75; **L** 93; **Sw** 113

scapular spine, **H** 5; **O** 35, 37, 39; **S** 57; **G** 75; **L** 93; **Sw** 113

scleral, **C** 131

sesamoid

distal, **H** 5, 8; **O** 35; **S** 57; **G** 75; **Sw** 113

hypotarsal, **C** 131

metatarsal, **Sw** 113

proximal, **H** 5, 8; **O** 35; **S** 57; **G** 75, 79; **L** 93; **Sw** 113

sphenoid, **H** 14; **L** 99; **Sw** 118

splint. *See* **H** 5, second and fourth metacarpal and metatarsal bones

sternum, **H** 5; **O** 35, 39, 45; **S** 57, 61; **G** 75, 81; **Sw** 113, 122; **C** 131, 134, 135

caudolateral process, **C** 131, 134

keel, **C** 131, 134

manubrium, **H** 5; **O** 35

thoracic process, **C** 131, 134, 135

xiphoid process, **H** 5; **O** 35, 44; **S** 57

talus, **H** 5; **O** 35; **S** 57; **G** 75; **Sw** 113

tarsal, **H** 5; **O** 35; **S** 57; **G** 75; **L** 93, 97; **Sw** 113

tarsometatarsal, **C** 131, 132

temporal, **H** 5; **O** 35; **S** 57; **G** 75, 82; **L** 93, 102; **Sw** 119; **C** 131

external acoustic meatus, **H** 5, 13; **O** 45; **G** 85; **C** 131

temporal fossa, **O** 38; **G** 75

zygomatic arch, **H** 13

tibia, **H** 5; **O** 35; **S** 57; **G** 75; **L** 93; **Sw** 113

lateral condyle, **O** 35; **S** 57; **G** 75; **L** 93

lateral malleolus, **O** 35; **S** 57; **G** 75; **L** 93

medial malleolus, **S** 57; **G** 75; **L** 93

tibiotarsal, **C** 131, 134, 135

ulna, **H** 5; **O** 35; **S** 57; **G** 75; **L** 93; **Sw** 113; **C** 131

olecranon, **H** 5; **G** 75

olecranon tuber, **H** 2, 5, 10; **O** 32, 35; **S** 57; **G** 75; **L** 93; **Sw** 113

vertebrae, **H** 5; **O** 35; **S** 57; **G** 75; **L** 93; **Sw** 113; **C** 131

caudal, **O** 47; **S** 57, 67; **G** 75; **L** 93; **Sw** 113, 117, 122, 125; **C** 131, 134, 136, 138, 139

cervical, **O** 44; **S** 57, 64; **G** 75; **L** 93, 101, 104; **Sw** 113, 122; **C** 131, 138, 139

lumbar, **O** 44, 46, 47; **S** 57, 63, 64, 66, 67; **G** 75, 86, 87; **L** 93, 104, 105, 106, 107; **Sw** 113, 117, 122, 124, 125

spinous process, **O** 35

transverse process, **O** 35

sacral. *See* sacrum

thoracic, **H** 5, 20; **O** 44; **S** 57, 63, 64; **G** 75; **L** 93, 104, 105; **Sw** 17, 122; **C** 131, 138, 139

vomer, **O** 40

Interdigital cleft, **G** 72
Internal inguinal ring, **H** 22; **O** 46; **G** 86; **L** 106
Intervertebral disc, **H** 13
Intestines. *See* Cecum, Colon, Duodenum, Ileum,
    Jejunum, Rectum
Ischiatic tuber, *See* Bone(s)

J

Jaw, **H** 3; **O** 33
Jejunum, **H** 13, 16; **O** 38, 39, 41, 42; **S** 60, 61; **G** 80, 81; **L**
    96, 97, 103; **Sw** 116, 117, 120; **C** 136
Joint(s)
    ankle, **H** 2; **C** 135
    antebrachiocarpal, **H** 13; **O** 39; **S** 61; **G** 81; **L** 97; **Sw**
        117
    atlantoaxial, **H** 5
    atlanto-occipital, **H** 5; **S** 64; **G** 81; **L** 97
    break joint, **S** 56
    carpometacarpal, **H** 13; **O** 39; **S** 61; **G** 81; **L** 97; **Sw** 117
    coffin, **H** 8, 13; **O** 39; **S** 61; **G** 81
    costovertebral, **H** 5, 13; **O** 39; **Sw** 117
    coxal, **H** 13; **O** 39; **G** 81; **L** 97; **Sw** 117; **C** 135
    cubital, **O** 39; **L** 97
    distal interphalangeal, **H** 13; **O** 39; **S** 61; **G** 81; **L** 97;
        Sw 117
    elbow, **H** 13; **O** 39; **S** 61; **G** 81; **L** 97; **Sw** 117
    femoropatellar, **H** 13; **O** 39; **S** 61; **G** 81; **L** 97; **Sw** 117
    femorotibial, **H** 11, 13; **O** 39; **S** 61, 64; **G** 81; **L** 97; **Sw**
        117; **C** 135
        fetlock, **H** 8, 13; **O** 39; **S** 61; **G** 81; **L** 97
    hip, **H** 13; **O** 39; **S** 61; **G** 81; **L** 97; **Sw** 117; **C** 135
    humeroradial, **H** 13
    humeroulnar, **H** 13
    intertarsal, **H** 13; **O** 39; **S** 61; **G** 81; **L** 97; **Sw** 117
    metacarpophalangeal, **H** 13; **O** 39; **S** 61; **G** 81; **L** 97;
        Sw 117
    metatarsophalangeal, **H** 13; **O** 39; **S** 61; **G** 81; **L** 97;
        Sw 117
    middle carpal, **H** 13; **O** 39; **S** 61; **G** 81; **L** 97; **Sw** 117
    pastern, **H** 8, 13; **O** 39; **S** 61; **G** 81
    proximal interphalangeal, **H** 8, 13; **O** 39; **S** 61; **G** 81;
        L 97; **Sw** 117

sacroiliac, **H** 13; **S** 61; **G** 81; **L** 97; **Sw** 117
scapulohumeral, **H** 13
shoulder, **H** 13; **O** 39; **S** 61; **G** 81; **L** 97; **Sw** 117; **C** 135
sternocostal, **H** 13
stifle, **H** 13; **O** 39; **S** 61; **G** 81; **L** 97; **Sw** 117
tarsocrural, **H** 13; **O** 39; **S** 61; **G** 81; **L** 97; **Sw** 117
tarsometatarsal, **H** 13; **O** 39; **S** 61; **G** 81; **L** 97; **Sw** 117
temporomandibular, **H** 13; **G** 81; **L** 97; **Sw** 117
wrist (carpal), **C** 133
Joint capsule
    coffin, **H** 8
    fetlock, **H** 8
    pastern, **H** 8
Jowl, **H** 3; **O** 33; **Sw** 110, 111, 112
Jugular groove, **H** 2, 3; **O** 32, 33; **G** 73

K

Kidneys, **H** 19, 20, 21; **O** 38, 44; **S** 60, 64, 65; **G** 80; **L** 96,
    104, 105; **Sw** 116, 117, 122, 123; **C** 138, 139, 140
Knee, **H** 2; **O** 32, 33; **S** 54, 55; **G** 72; **L** 90; **Sw** 110, 111; **C**
    129

L

Labial vestibule, **Sw** 118
Lacertus fibrosus, **H** 10
Larynx, **H** 13, 14; **Sw** 117
    laryngeal ventricle, **H** 14
Lateral ala, **H** 2
Left flank incision
Leg, **H** 2; **O** 32; **S** 54; **G** 72; **L** 90, 91; **Sw** 111; **C** 129
    "Leg" of lamb, **S** 54, 56
Ligament(s)
    accessory l. of deep digital flexor m., **H** 10
    accessory l. of superficial digital flexor m., **H** 10
    broad l. of uterus, **S** 67, 69; **L** 107; **Sw** 125
    broad sacrotuberal, **H** 12, 13; **O** 38, 39; **S** 61; **G** 81; **L**
        97; **Sw** 116
    carpal check, **H** 10
    collateral sesamoidean, **H** 8
    digital anular, **G** 78
    distal digital anular, **H** 12

distal sesamoidean, **H** 10, 11

distal sesamoidean impar, **H** 8

dorsal l. of tarsus, **O** 37; **G** 77

interdigital, **G** 78

middle l. of bladder, **H** 24; **G** 86; **Sw** 124

nephrosplenic, **H** 19

nuchal, **H** 13, 14, 21; **O** 39, 40; **S** 61; **G** 81, 83; **L** 95, 96, 97, 99, 105

palmar anular, **H** 8

radial check, **H** 10

supraspinous, **H** 21; **O** 38, 39; **S** 61; **G** 81; **L** 96, 97

suspensory (interosseus medius m.), **H** 7, 10, 11; **O** 37; **S** 59; **G** 77; **L** 95, 98

"T", **H** 7

triangular l. of liver, **H** 21

ventral l. of oviduct, **C** 141

Linea alba, **G** 86; **L** 106

Lingual fossa. *See* Tongue

Lips, **H** 14; **O** 40; **G** 73, 83; **L** 99; **Sw** 110, 118

Liver, **H** 12, 20, 21, 24; **O** 38, 42, 43, 44; **S** 60; **G** 80, 84; **L** 96, 104; **Sw** 116, 117, 122, 123; **C** 134, 135

    caudate process of caudate lobe, **O** 44

    left lobe, **H** 21; **O** 44

    quadrate lobe, **H** 20; **O** 44

    right lobe, **H** 20; **O** 44; **L** 104

Loin, **H**2; **O** 32; **S** 54.56; **G** 72; **L** 90; **Sw** 110, 111, 112

Lower foreshank, **S** 54, 56

Lower hindshank, **S** 54, 56

Lumbosacral plexus. *See* Nerve(s)

Lung, **H** 12, 13; **O** 38, 39, 40; **S** 60, 61; **G** 80, 81; **L** 96, 97; **Sw** 116, 117; **C** 134, 135, 137

Lymph node(s)

    axillary, **H** 27; **O** 51; **Sw** 121

    caudal deep cervical, **H** 27; **O** 51; **Sw** 121

    caudal mediastinal, **O** 45; **S** 65; **G** 84, 5

    caudal mesenteric, **H** 27

    cranial deep cervical, **H** 27, **O** 51; **Sw** 121

    deep inguinal, **H** 27

    dorsal thoracic, **H** 27

    epigastric, **O** 51

    gluteal, **O** 51; **Sw** 121

    intercostal, **O** 51

    lateral iliac, **O** 51; **Sw** 121

    lateral retropharyngeal, **H** 27; **O** 38, 51, 56; **Sw** 121

    lumbar aortic and renal, **H** 27; **O** 51; **Sw** 121

    mandibular, **H** 27; **O** 51; **S** 62; **Sw** 121

    medial iliac, **H** 27; **O** 51; **Sw** 121

    medial retropharyngeal, **H** 27; **O** 51; **Sw** 121

    mediastinal, **H** 27; **L** 104; **Sw** 121

    mesenteric, **H** 27; **O** 51; **Sw** 121

    middle deep cervical, **H** 27; **O** 51; **Sw** 121

    parotid, **H** 27; **O** 51; **Sw** 121

    popliteal, **H** 27; **O** 51; **Sw** 121

        deep, **Sw** 121

        superficial, **Sw** 121

    sacral, **H** 27; **Sw** 121

    sternal, **O** 51; **Sw** 121

    subiliac, **H** 7, 27; **O** 36, 51; **G** 77; **L** 93; **Sw** 114, 121

    superficial cervical, **H** 27; **O** 38, 51; **L** 101

        dorsal, **Sw** 121

        ventral, **Sw** 121

    superficial inguinal, **H** 27; **O** 39, 51; **S** 66, 67; **G** 81, 84; **L** 106, 107; **Sw** 121, 124, 125

    supramammary, **O** 39, 51; **L** 107; **Sw** 121

    thoracic aortic, **Sw** 121

    tracheobronchial, **H** 27; **O** 51

    ventral thoracic, **H** 27

Lymph vessels, **H** 27; **O** 51

    chyle cistern, **H** 27; **O** 51

    intestinal trunk, **H** 27; **O** 51; **Sw** 121

    left tracheal trunk, **O** 51; **Sw** 121

    lumbar trunk, **H** 27; **O** 51; **Sw** 121

    right tracheal trunk, **H** 27

    thoracic duct, **H** 27; **O** 51; **Sw** 121

M

Mammary glands. *See* Gland(s) and Udder

Mane, **H** 3

Manica flexoria, **L** 98

Manus (hand), **H** 3; **C** 128

Meatus, dorsal, middle, ventral, **H** 14; **O** 40; **G** 83; **L** 99; **Sw** 118

Medial canthus, **O** 32

Mesocolon, **G** 87

Mesometrium **H** 23; **O** 47

Mesosalpinx, **H** 23; **S** 69

Mesovarium, **H** 23; **O** 47; **S** 67, 69

Metacarpal tuberosity, **H** 10. *See* Bone(s)

Metacarpus, **H** 2; **O** 32, 33; **S** 54; **G** 72; **L** 90; **Sw** 111

Metatarsal cushion, **C** 128

Metatarsus, **H** 2; **O** 33; **S** 54; **G** 72; **L** 90; **Sw** 111

Milk well, **O** 33

Muscle(s)

accessory patagial, **C** 133

adductor, **O** 46; **S** 60; **G** 80; **L** 96, 106; **Sw** 116, 124, 125

ascending pectoral, **H** 7; **O** 37; **S** 59; **G** 77; **L** 95; **Sw** 115

biceps brachii, **H** 7; **O** 38; **S** 60; **G** 80; **L** 96; **Sw** 116; **C** 133

biceps femoris, **H** 7; **Sw** 115; **C** 132, 133

biventer. *See* Semispinalis capitis, **Sw** 117; **C** 132–135

brachialis, **H** 7; **O** 37; **S** 59, 60; **G** 77, 80; **L** 95, 96; **Sw** 115, 116

brachiocephalicus, **H** 7; **O** 38; **S** 59, 62; **L** 95, 101; **Sw** 115

buccinator, **H** 7; **O** 37; **S** 59; **G** 77; **L** 95; **Sw** 115

bulbospongiosus, **H** 20; **O** 46; **G** 84, 86; **L** 106; **Sw** 124

bulbourethral,**Sw** 124

caninus, **H** 7; **O** 36; **Sw** 115

caudal capital oblique, **H** 12, 13; **O** 46; **S** 61; **G** 81; **L** 97

caudal preputial, **O** 36; **Sw** 114

caudal scapulohumeral, **C** 133

cloacal elevator, **C** 132, 133

cloacal sphincter, **C** 132, 133, 135

coccygeus, **O** 37; **S** 60; **G** 80

coccygeus lateralis, **C** 132, 133

common digital extensor, **H** 7, 10; **O** 37; **S** 59; **G** 77; **L** 95; **Sw** 115

complexus. *See* Semispinalis capitis, **Sw** 117; **C** 132–135

cranial capital oblique, **H** 13; **O** 39; **S** 61; **G** 81; **L** 96, 97; **Sw** 116, 117

cranial preputial, **O** 36; **Sw** 114

cranial tibial, **H** 7, 12; **O** 37; **S** 59; **L** 95; **Sw** 115

cutaneus colli, **H** 6; **O** 36; **S** 58; **G** 76; **L** 93; **Sw** 114; **C** 132

cutaneus faciei, **H** 6; **O** 36; **S** 58; **G** 76; **L** 93; **Sw** 114

cutaneus nasi, **G** 76

cutaneus trunci, **H** 6; **O** 36; **S** 58, 63; **G** 76; **L** 93; **Sw** 114

deep digital flexor, **H** 7, 10, 12; **O** 37, 38; **S** 59, 60; **G** 77, 80; **L** 95, 96; **Sw** 115, 116; **C** 133

deltoideus, **H** 7; **O** 37; **S** 59, 60; **G** 77, 80; **L** 95, 96; **Sw** 115; **C** 132

depressor labii inferioris, **H** 7; **S** 59; **G** 77; **Sw** 115

depressor labii superioris, **H** 7; **Sw** 115

depressor mandibulae, **C** 132

depressor palpebrae, **G** 77; **Sw** 115

descending pectoral, **H** 7; **O** 37; **G** 77; **L** 95

digastricus, **H** 12, 13

dilator naris, **H** 14

dorsal capital straight, **H** 14; **O** 39; **S** 61, **G** 81, 83; **L** 97, 99, **Sw** 119

dorsal interosseous, **C** 132

extensor carpi obliquus, **H** 7, 12; **O** 37; **S** 59; **G** 77; **L** 95; **Sw** 115

extensor carpi radialis, **H** 7, 10; **O** 37; **S** 59; **G** 77; **L** 95; **Sw** 115

extensor metacarpi radialis, **C** 132, 133

external abdominal oblique, **H** 7; **O** 37; **S** 59, 63; **G** 77; **L** 95; **Sw** 115; **C** 132, 133

external anal sphincter, **H** 20, 21; **S** 66; **Sw** 124

external mandibular adductor, **C** 132

fifth digital extensor, **Sw** 115

flexor carpi radialis, **H** 7, 10; **O** 37; **S** 59; **G** 77; **L** 95; **Sw** 115

flexor carpi ulnaris, **H** 7; **S** 59; **G** 77; **C** 133

flexor perforans and perforatus, **C** 132

frontalis, **O** 36, 37; **S** 59; **G** 77; **L** 95

frontoscutularis, **H** 6

gastrocnemius, **H** 7, 12; **O** 37, 38; **S** 59, 60; **G** 77, 80; **L** 95, 96; **Sw** 115, 116; **C** 132, 133

genioglossus, **H** 14; **G** 83; **L** 99; **Sw** 118

geniohyoideus, **H** 14; **G** 83; **L** 99; **Sw** 118

gluteobiceps, **O** 37; **S** 59; **G** 77; **L** 95

gracilis, **O** 46; **Sw** 124

hyoepiglottic, **H** 14

iliacus, **H** 12; **O** 38

iliocostalis thoracis, **H** 12; **O** 38; **S** 60; **G** 80; **L** 96; **Sw** 115, 116

infraspinatus, **H** 12; **O** 38; **S** 60; **G** 80; **L** 96

internal abdominal oblique, **H** 22; **O** 37, 47; **S** 59, 63, 66; **G** 77; **L** 95, 107

interosseus medius, **H** 10; **O** 36; **G** 78
    See also Suspensory ligament, **H** 7, 10, 11; **O** 37; **S** 59; **G** 77; **L** 95, 98

interosseus secundus, **L** 98

intertransversarii, **H** 12, 13; **O** 39; **S** 60, 61, 62; **G** 81; **L** 95, 96, 97; **Sw** 116, 117

intertransversarius longus, **O** 38; **S** 61; **G** 81; **L** 97

ischiocavernosus, **O** 46; **S** 64, 66; **G** 84, 86; **L** 104, 106; **Sw** 124

lateral digital extensor, **H** 7, 10, 12; **O** 37; **S** 59; **G** 77; **L** 95; **Sw** 115

latissimus dorsi, **H** 7; **O** 37; **S** 59; **G** 77; **L** 95; **Sw** 115; **C** 132, 133

levator ani, **C** 132, 133

levator coccygeus, **C** 132, 133

levator labii superioris, **H** 7; **O** 36; **Sw** 115

levator nasolabialis, **H** 7; **O** 36; **S** 59; **G** 77; **L** 95; **Sw** 115

long digital extensor, **H** 7, 12; **O** 37; **S** 59; **G** 77; **L** 95

long patagial tensor, **C** 132, 133

longissimus atlantis, **H** 12; **O** 38; **S** 60; **G** 80; **L** 95; **Sw** 116, 117

longissimus capitis, **H** 12; **O** 38; **S** 60; **G** 80; **L** 95, 96; **Sw** 116, 117

longissimus cervicis, **H** 12; **O** 38; **S** 60; **G** 80; **L** 95, 96; **Sw** 117

longissimus thoracis and lumborum, **H** 12; **O** 38; **S** 60; **G** 80; **L** 96; **Sw** 116

longus atlantis, **L** 96

longus capitis, **H** 12, 14; **S** 60; **G** 80; **L** 96, 99; **Sw** 116, 117

longus coli, **H** 12, 14; **S** 61, 62; **G** 81, 83; **L** 97, 99, 101; **C** 133, 134, 135

major long digital flexor, **C** 133

malaris, **O** 37; **S** 59; **G** 77

masseter, **H** 7; **O** 37; **S** 59, 62; **G** 77; **L** 95; **Sw** 115

mentalis, **H** 14; **Sw** 115

middle gluteal, **H** 7, 19; **O** 37, 38; **S** 59, 60; **G** 77, 80; **L** 95, 96; **Sw** 115, 116

multifidus cervicis, **H** 13; **O** 39; **S** 61; **G** 80, 81; **L** 97

mylohyoideus, **O** 37

obturator internis, **H** 23; **O** 46, 47

occipital hyoideus, **H** 12

omohyoideus, **H** 7, 14; **S** 62

omotransversarius, **H** 7; **O** 37; **S** 59; **G** 77; **L** 95; **Sw** 115

orbicularis oris, **Sw** 115

parotidoauricularis, **H** 7; **S** 59, 62; **G** 77; **L** 95

peroneus longus, **O** 37; **S** 59; **G** 77; **L** 95; **Sw** 115; **C** 132, 133

peroneus tertius, **H** 7, 11; **O** 37; **S** 59; **G** 77; **L** 95; **Sw** 115

platysma, **Sw** 114

psoas major, **O** 38; **Sw** 116

quadratus lumborum, **Sw** 116

quadriceps femoris, **H** 11, 12

rectus abdominis, **H** 22; **S** 66, 67; **G** 86, 87; **L** 106, 107; **Sw** 124, 125

rectus femoris, **H** 12; **O** 38; **S** 60; **G** 80; **L** 96; **Sw** 116

retractor penis, **H** 20; **O** 44, 46; **S** 64, 66; **G** 84, 86; **L** 106; **Sw** 124

rhomboideus, **H** 7, 12; **O** 38; **S** 60; **G** 80; **L** 96; **Sw** 116; **C** 134

sacrocaudalis, **O** 37

sartorius, **C** 132, 133

scalenus, **H** 12; **O** 38, 39; **S** 60; **G** 80; **L** 96, 101

scutularis, **O** 36

semimembranosus, **H** 7, 12; **O** 38; **S** 59, 60; **G** 80; **L** 95, 96; **Sw** 115, 116; **C** 132, 133

semispinalis capitis, **H** 12; **S** 60; **G** 80; **Sw** 117, 118
    biventer cervicis, **Sw** 117; **C** 132, 133, 134, 135
    complexus, **Sw** 117; **C** 132–135

semitendinosus, **H** 7, 12; **O** 37, 38; **S** 59, 60; **G** 80; **L** 95, 96; **Sw** 115; **C** 132, 133

serratus dorsalis caudalis, **H** 7; **O** 35

serratus dorsalis cranialis, **G** 77; **L** 95

serratus superficialis, **C** 133

serratus ventralis, **H** 7; **O** 37; **S** 59; **G** 77; **L** 95, 96; **Sw** 115, 116

short digital extensor, **H** 12; **Sw** 115

Muscle(s)—*Continued*

    soleus, **H** 7, 15; **O** 38; **S** 60; **Sw** 116

    spinalis cervicis, **H** 13

    spinalis thoracis, **H** 12

    splenius, **H** 7; **O** 38; **L** 95, 96; **Sw** 116

    sternocephalicus, **H** 7; **O** 37, 38; **S** 59; **G** 77; **L** 95, 101, 104; **Sw** 115, 116

    sternohyoideus, **H** 14; **O** 38; **S** 60, 62; **G** 80; **L** 95; **Sw** 115, 116, 118

    sternothyrohyoideus, **H** 10, 11, 13; **O** 38; **S** 60, 62; **G** 77, 80; **L** 95; **Sw** 116; **C** 132, 133, 134

    sternothyroideus, **O** 38

    subclavius, **H** 7; **Sw** 115

    superficial gluteal, **H** 7; **Sw** 115

    superficial pectoral, **C** 132, 133

    superficial pronator, **C** 133

    supraspinalis, **H** 12; **O** 38; **S** 60; **G** 80; **L** 96; **Sw** 115

    temporalis, **H** 7; **O** 38

    tensor fasciae antebrachii, **Sw** 115

    tensor fasciae latae, **H** 7, 11; **O** 37; **S** 59; **G** 77; **L** 95; **Sw** 115; **C** 132, 133

    teres minor, **H** 12

    thoracic and cervical spinalis and semispinalis, **O** 38, 39; **S** 60, 61; **G** 80, 81; **L** 96, 97; **Sw** 116

    transverse abdominal, **O** 47; **S** 63

    trapezius, **H** 7; **O** 37; **S** 59; **G** 77; **L** 95; **Sw** 115

    triceps brachii, **H** 7, 10; **O** 37; **S** 59; **G** 77; **L** 95; **Sw** 115; **C** 133

    ulnaris lateralis, **H** 7; **O** 37; **S** 59; **L** 95; **Sw** 115

    urethralis, **H** 22; **O** 46; **S** 66; **G** 84; **L** 104, 106; **Sw** 124

    vastus lateralis, **H** 12; **O** 38; **S** 60; **G** 80; **L** 96; **Sw** 116

    zygomaticoauricularis, **S** 59; **G** 77; **L** 95

    zygomaticus, **H** 7; **O** 37; **S** 59; **G** 77; **L** 95; **Sw** 115

Muzzle, **H** 3; **O** 32; **S** 54; **G** 72; **L** 90

    nasolabial plane of, **O** 33

N

Nasal septum, **H** 14; **L** 99

Navicular bursa, **H** 8

Neck, **H** 2; **O** 32; **S** 54, 56; **G** 72; **L** 90; **Sw** 111

Nerve(s)

    accessory, **H** 28; **O** 50

axillary, **H** 28; **O** 50

brachial plexus, **H** 28; **O** 50

caudal cutaneous antebrachial, **H** 28; **O** 50

caudal cutaneous sural, **H** 28

caudal laryngeal, **S** 62

caudal rectal, **H** 28

cervical, **H** 28; **O** 50; **S** 62

common peroneal, **H** 28; **O** 36, 38, 50

communicating branch, **H** 28

cornual branch of lacrimal, **G** 82

cranial gluteal, **O** 50

deep peroneal, **H** 28; **O** 50

dorsal br. of lateral palmar digital, **H** 28

dorsal br. of lateral plantar digital, **H** 28

dorsal common digital II, III, & IV, **G** 78; **L** 98

dorsal digital, **O** 58

dorsal proper (abaxial & axial) digital III & IV, **G** 78; **L** 98

dorsal spinal, **H** 28; **O** 50

facial, **H** 7, 28, 29; **O** 37, 50; **G** 77; **Sw** 115

femoral, **H** 28; **O** 50

genitofemoral, **H** 28; **O** 50

glossopharyngeal, **H** 29

ilioinguinal, **H** 28; **O** 50

infraorbital, **H** 7, 28; **O** 50

infratrochlear, cornual br. & frontal br., **G** 82

intercostal, **H** 28; **O** 50

lateral cutaneous antebrachial, **H** 28

lateral cutaneous femoral, **H** 28

lateral dorsal metatarsal, **H** 28

lateral palmar, **H** 28

lateral palmar digital, **H** 28

lateral plantar, **H** 28

lateral plantar digital, **H** 28

lateral thoracic, **H** 28; **O** 50

long thoracic, **H** 28; **O** 50

lumbosacral plexus, **H** 28; **O** 50

mandibular, **H** 28; **O** 50

mandibular alveolar, **H** 28

maxillary, **O** 50

medial cutaneous antebrachial, **H** 28; **O** 50

medial dorsal metatarsal, **H** 28

Penis—*Continued*
    spongy tubercle, **S** 68
Peritoneal cavity, **S** 63
Peritoneum. *See* Serosa, **S** 63
Pes, **H** 2
Phallic bodies. *See* Cloaca
Pharynx, **C** 136
    laryngopharynx, **O** 40; **G** 83; **L** 99; **Sw** 118
    nasopharynx, **H** 14; **O** 40; **G** 83; **L** 99; **Sw** 118
    oropharynx, **H** 14; **O** 40; **G** 83; **L** 99; **Sw** 118
    pharyngeal recess, **Sw** 118
    pharyngeal septum, **O** 40; **G** 83
    pharyngeal tonsil, **G** 83
Pin, **O** 32
Pinna, **H** 3; **O** 32, 33; **S** 54, 59; **G** 72, 73; **L** 90, 91
Point
    of elbow, **H** 2; **O** 32; **G** 73; **L** 91; **Sw** 110
    of hip, **H** 3; **Sw** 111
    of hock, **H** 3; **O** 33; **S** 55; **G** 73; **L** 91; **Sw** 110
    of shoulder, **H** 2; **O** 32; **G** 73; **L** 91; **Sw** 111
Poll, **H** 2; **O** 32, 33; **G** 72, 73; **L** 90; **Sw** 111
Pouch(es)
    cutaneous, **S** 54, 55
    guttural, **H** 14
Preen gland. *See* Gland(s), uropygial
Prepuce, **H** 2, 22; **S** 54, 68; **G** 76, 86; **L** 106; **Sw** 110, 114, 124
    external (sheath), **H** 22
    internal, **H** 22; **S** 68
    preputial diverticulum, **Sw** 114, 124
    preputial orifice, **O** 32; **S** 124
Proctodeum. *See* Cloaca
Propatagium, **C** 128, 129
Proventriculus, **C** 135, 136, 138, 139
Pygostyle. *See* Bone(s)
Pylorus. *See* Stomach

Q

Quarter, **H** 2

R

Rack, **S** 56
Reciprocal apparatus, **H** 11
Rectum, **H** 16, 20, 21, 23; **O** 41, 45, 46, 47; **S** 61, 65, 66, 67; **G** 80, 84, 86, 87; **L** 103, 105, 106, 107; **Sw** 117, 123, 124, 125; **C** 134, 136, 138, 139, 140, 141
    ampulla, **H** 23
    transverse plicae, **H** 22
Reticulum, **O** 39, 41, 43, 45; **S** 64, 65; **G** 85
Rib margin. *See* Bone(s)
Round, **O** 32
Rumen, **O** 39, 42, 43, 45; **S** 60, 61, 63, 64, 65; **G** 81, 84, 85
    interior, **O** 41; **S** 63
Rump, **O** 32; **S** 54; **G** 72; **L** 90; **Sw** 110

S

Saddle, **C** 128, 130
Scrotum, **H** 22; **O** 32, 38; **S** 54, 66; **G** 86; **L** 106; **Sw** 110, 114
    seminal vesicle. *See* Gland(s)
    tunica albuginea, **S** 58; **G** 76
Serosa of rumen, **S** 63
Shank, **C** 128, 129
Shoulder, **H** 3; **O** 32; **S** 54, 56; **G** 72; **L** 90; **Sw** 110; **C** 128, 129
Sinus
    frontal, **H** 14; **O** 40; **G** 83, 84; **L** 99; **Sw** 118
    cornual diverticulum, **O** 44; **G** 84
    sphenoid, **H** 14; **Sw** 118
Skin & subcutis, **S** 63; **G** 79
Slipper, **L** 91, 98
Snout, **Sw** 110, 111
Spermatic cord, **H** 22; **Sw** 122, 124
Spinal cord, **H** 14, 28, 29; **O** 50; **G** 83; **L** 99; **Sw** 118
Spleen, **H** 13, 19, 21; **O** 39, 43, 45, 51; **S** 61; **G** 81; **L** 97; **Sw** 117, 123; **C** 138, 139
Spur, **C** 128
Stay apparatus
    forelimb, **H** 10
    hindlimb, **H** 11
Sternocoracoclavicular membrane, **C** 134

Stifle, **H** 2, 11; **O** 32; **S** 61; **G** 81; **L** 97; **Sw** 110

Stomach, **H** 16, 21; **L** 96, 97, 103, 104, 105;
    Sw 116, 117, 120, 122, 123
    diverticulum ventriculi, **Sw** 120
    gastric compartments, **L** 96, 97, 103, 104, 105
    proper gastric gland region, **L** 103, 104
    pyloric antrum, **H** 16
    pylorus, **G** 80; **Sw** 120

Suburethral diverticulum. *See* Urethra

Supraglenoid tubercle. *See* Bone(s), scapula

Switch, **O** 32

Synsacrum. *See* Bone(s)

T

Tail head, **H** 2; **O** 32, 33; **G** 72; **L** 90; **Sw** 110

Tarsometatarsus, **C** 129

Tarsus, **H** 2; **O** 32; **S** 54; **G** 72; **L** 90; **Sw** 111

Teat(s) **H** 3; **O** 33, 45, 47; **S** 67; **G** 73; **L** 97, 105, 107
    streak canal (papillary duct), **O** 45, 47; **S** 65, 67; **G** 85, 87
    teat sinus, **O** 45; **S** 65, 67; **G** 85, 87

Tendon(s)
    biceps brachii m., **H** 10
    common calcaneal, **H** 7
    common digital extensor m., **H** 7, 8, 10; **G** 78, 79; **L** 95, 98
    cranial tibial m., **H** 7; **O** 37; **S** 59
    cunean, **H** 7
    deep digital flexor m., **H** 7, 8, 10; **O** 37, 38; **S** 59, 60; **G** 77, 78, 79, 80; **L** 95, 98
    extensor carpi obliquus m., **H** 7; **O** 36, 37; **G** 77
    gastrocnemius m., **S** 56
    gastrocnemius + digital flexor mm., **C** 132, 133
    lateral digital extensor m., **H** 7; **G** 78; **L** 95, 98
    long digital extensor m., **H** 7; **O** 37; **S** 59; **G** 77; **L** 95; **C** 132
    peroneus longus m., **S** 59
    peroneus tertius m., **H** 7, 10
    superficial digital flexor m., **H** 7, 8, 10, 13; **O** 37, 38; **S** 59, 60; **G** 77, 78, 79, 80; **L** 95, 98
    symphyseal, **H** 22; **O** 47; **S** 66, 67; **G** 86, 87; **L** 106, 107; **Sw** 124, 125

Testis, **H** 20, 22; **O** 44, 46; **S** 64, 66; **G** 84, 86; **L** 104, 106; **Sw** 122, 124; **C** 138, 140
    tunica albuginea, **Sw** 116

Thigh, **H** 2; **S** 54, 55; **G** 72; **L** 90, 91; **Sw** 111

Throatlatch, **H** 2

Thymus, **H** 24; **O** 51; **Sw** 117

Toe Nails, **L** 90, 91, 98

Tongue, **H** 14; **O** 40; **G** 83; **L** 99; **Sw** 118; **C** 136
    lingual fossa, **O** 40; **G** 83

Tonsil
    palatine, **O** 40
    pharyngeal, **O** 40

Tooth (teeth)
    canine, **H** 12, 15; **G** 82; **L** 102; **Sw** 119
    cement, **H** 15
    cheek, **G** 84
    crown, **H** 15
    cup, **H** 15
    dental star, **H** 15
    dentin, **H** 15
    enamel, **H** 15
    incisor, **H** 13, 14, 15, 24; **O** 39, 44; **S** 60; **G** 80, 82, 84; **L** 102, 105; **Sw** 119
    infundibulum, **H** 15
    molar, **H** 15; **O** 44; **G** 82; **L** 102; **Sw** 119
    occlusal surface, **H** 15
    points, **H** 15
    premolar, **H** 15; **O** 44; **G** 82; **L** 102; **Sw** 119
    pulp cavity of, **H** 15
    root, **H** 15
    wolf, **H** 13, 15

Topline, **O** 32; **S** 54

Trachea, **H** 13, 14; **O** 39, 40; **S** 60, 61, 62; **G** 80, 81, 83; **L** 96, 97, 101; **Sw** 117, **C** 132, 134

U

Udder, **H** 21; **O** 33, 39, 45; **S** 65, 67; **G** 73, 77, 81; **L** 107
    forequarters, **O** 33, 47; **L** 107
    gland sinus, **O** 45; **S** 65, 67; **G** 85, 87
    hindquarters, **O** 33, 47; **L** 107
    suspensory apparatus, **O** 45, 47

Umbilicus, **H** 24

Umbilicus—*Continued*
    umbilical cord, **H** 24
Uncinate process. *See* Bone(s), ribs
Urachus, **H** 24
Ureters, **H** 20, 21, 22, 24; **O** 44, 46; **S** 64, 65; **G** 84, 86; **L**
    104, 105, 106; **Sw** 122, 123, 124, 125; **C** 136, 138,
    140, 141
    openings, **C** 140, 141
Urethra, **H** 22, 23, 24; **O** 46; **S** 67, 68; **G** 85, 87; **L** 107; **Sw**
    123, 125
    dorsal diverticulum, **O** 46
    external urethral orifice, **H** 22; **S** 67, 69
    pelvic, **H** 22; **O** 46; **G** 86; **L** 106
    penile, **H** 22; **O** 46
    suburethral diverticulum, **O** 47; **S** 67; **L** 107; **Sw** 125
    urethral papilla, **O** 47
Urinary bladder, **H** 20, 21, 22, 23, 24; **O** 39, 45, 46, 47;
    S 64, 65, 66, 67; **G** 84, 85, 86, 87; **L** 104, 105, 106,
    107; **Sw** 116, 117, 122, 124, 125
Urodeum. *See* Cloaca
Uterine tube(s), **H** 21, 23; **S** 69; **G** 87; **L** 105, 107; **Sw** 125
    infundibulum, **H** 23; **O** 47
      fimbriae, **S** 69
Uterus, **H** 21, 23; **O** 39, 45; **S** 65, 69; **G** 85; **L** 105; **Sw** 123
    body, **H** 21, 23; **O** 47; **S** 67, 69; **G** 87; **L** 107; **Sw** 123, 125
    uterine cervix, **H** 23; **O** 47; **S** 67, 69; **G** 87; **L** 107; **Sw**
      125
      cervical canal, **H** 23
      external os, **H** 23; **O** 47
    uterine horns (cornua), **H** 21, 23; **O** 47; **S** 67, 69;
      G 85, 87; **L** 107; **Sw** 123, 125

V

Vagina, **H** 21, 23; **O** 45, 47; **S** 65, 67, 69; **G** 85, 87; **L** 105;
    Sw 117, 123, 125
    proper, **H** 23; **O** 47; **S** 67; **G** 87; **L** 106
    vestibule, **H** 23; **O** 47; **S** 67, 69; **G** 87; **L** 106; **Sw** 125
Veins
    angularis oculi, **O** 48; **G** 77
    axillary, **H** 26; **O** 48
    azygous, **H** 20, 26; **O** 44, 45, 48; **G** 84, 85; **L** 105; **Sw**
      123

brachial, **H** 26; **O** 48
buccal, **H** 26
caudal auricular, **H** 26
caudal br. of medial saphenous, **H** 26
caudal epigastric, **H** 26; **O** 48
caudal femoral, **H** 26
caudal gluteal, **H** 26
caudal superficial epigastric, **H** 26; **O** 37, 48
caudal tibial, **H** 26
caudal vena cava, **H** 20, 21, 26; **O** 44, 45, 48; **S** 64, 65;
    G 84, 85; **L** 104; **Sw** 122, 123; **C** 138, 139
cephalic, **H** 7, 26; **O** 37, 48; **S** 59; **G** 77
circumflex femoral, **O** 48
collateral ulnar, **H** 26; **O** 48
costocervical trunk, **H** 26; **O** 48
cranial br. of lateral saphenous, **O** 48
cranial br. of medial saphenous, **H** 26
cranial epigastric, **H** 26; **O** 37, 48
cranial gluteal, **H** 26
cranial superficial epigastric, **H** 26; **O** 48
cranial tibial, **H** 26; **O** 48
cranial vena cava, **H** 21, 26; **O** 44, 45, 48; **S** 64, 65; **G**
    84, 85; **L** 104, 105; **Sw** 122, 123
    left, **C** 135, 139
    right, **C** 134, 138
deep cervical, **H** 26
deep circumflex iliac, **H** 26; **O** 48
deep facial, **H** 26
deep femoral, **H** 26; **O** 48
digital, **H** 26
dorsal, **H** 26; **O** 48
dorsal common digital III, **H** 26; **O** 46; **L** 98
dorsal nasal, **H** 26; **O** 48; **G** 77
dorsal proper digital, **O** 48
dorsal scapular, **H** 26
external iliac, **H** 46; **O** 48
external jugular, **H** 7, 13, 26; **O** 37, 48; **S** 59, 65; **G** 77,
    84, 85
external pudendal, **H** 26; **O** 48
external thoracic, **H** 26; **O** 48
facial, **H** 7, 26; **O** 37; **G** 77

hepatic, **H** 26; **O** 48

iliolumbar, **H** 26

intercostal, **H** 26; **O** 48; **Sw** 123

internal iliac, **H** 26; **O** 48

internal jugular, **O** 48; **S** 62

internal thoracic, **H** 26; **O** 48

interosseous, **O** 48

jugular, **L** 95, 101, 104, 105; **C** 132, 133, 134, 135, 139

lateral auricular, **Sw** 114

lateral palmar, **H** 26

lateral plantar, **O** 48

lateral sacral, **H** 26

lateral saphenous, **H** 7, 26; **O** 37, 48; **S** 59; **G** 77

lateral thoracic, **H** 7; **Sw** 114

linguofacial, **H** 26; **G** 77

maxillary, **H** 26; **O** 48; **S** 62; **G** 77

medial plantar, **H** 26; **O** 48

medial saphenous, **H** 26; **O** 48; **S** 59; **G** 77

median, **H** 26; **O** 37, 48

median sacral, **O** 48

milk. *See* Subcutaneous abdominal, **O** 33, 36, 37; **G** 73, 77

occipital, **H** 26; **O** 48; **S** 62

ovarian, **H** 26

palmar common digital, **O** 48

palmar proper digital, **O** 48

pampiniform plexus, **O** 46; **S** 66; **G** 86; **L** 106

plantar common digital, **O** 48

plantar proper digital, **O** 48

popliteal, **O** 48

portal, **O** 48

prostatic, **H** 26; **O** 48

pudendal epigastric, **H** 26; **O** 48

pulmonary, **H** 25; **O** 45; **S** 65; **G** 85; **L** 105; **C** 138

renal, **H** 26; **O** 48

rostral auricular, **H** 26

subclavian, **H** 26; **O** 48; **S** 65; **G** 85

subcutaneous abdominal, **O** 33, 37; **G** 73, 77

subscapular, **H** 26; **O** 48

superficial cervical, **H** 26; **O** 48

superficial thoracic, **H** 26

testicular, **H** 22, 26; **O** 46, 48; **S** 66; **G** 86; **L** 106; **Sw** 124

thoracodorsal, **H** 26; **O** 48

transverse facial, **H** 26

umbilical, **H** 24

vertebral, **H** 26, **O** 48

Vent, **C** 132, 134, 135, 140

Ventriculus (gizzard), **C** 134, 135, 136, 138, 139

Vulva, **H** 13, 21, 23; **O** 45, 47; **S** 65; **G** 73, 77, 85; **L** 105; **Sw** 117, 123, 125

clitoris, **H** 23; **O** 47; **S** 67; **L** 107

vulvar labia, **H** 23; **O** 47; **S** 67, 69; **G** 87; **L** 107

W

Wattle(s), **G** 73; **C** 128, 129

Wing bar. *See* Feather(s)

Wing bow. *See* Feather(s)

Withers, **H** 2; **O** 32; **S** 54; **G** 72; **L** 90; **Sw** 111

Wrist joint. *See* Joint(s)

X

Xiphoid process. *See* Bone(s), sternum

Z

Zygomatic arch, **H** 13. *See also* Bone(s)